Praise for Love Nev

"This is a *real* book about what it's like to do the Alzheimer's caregiver job 24/7. It's clearly written so the lay person can understand and learn from it, yet full of introspective insights for the professional as well. I could relate it easily to other Alzheimer's families that I've had the privilege to serve. The issue of the abusive patient is so often not discussed and it needs to be known! I highly recommend this book (and already have to my co-workers). It will be so helpful to so many who are dealing with similar situations. I can see this book helping a lot of people and being a turning point for them. I strongly feel that *Love Never Sleeps* is invaluable to all those needing to make an educated and well-informed decision regarding home care versus nursing home placement. A well, well done book!"

—*Barbara Jensen, hospice R.N.*

"I believe that the real value of this book is that it offers emotional support to those faced with confronting Alzheimer's. It provides insights and experiences combined with knowledge of the disease gained from research into its effects and pathology. It's very important that people understand what the disease does, so they won't emotionally separate as caregivers, whether they make the difficult decision to care within the home or not. *Love Never Sleeps* depicts the experiences of three people facing Alzheimer's inside their own home. It is an invaluable guide to anyone confronting the agonizing difficulties of caring for a loved one progressing through the disease. It is written in a concise and honest manner with the problems both the patient and caregivers experience tied to the known clinical descriptions of Alzheimer's. It is a heartfelt gift of love from Mary, Sally, and Mary Belle herself to you and your loved ones."

—*William Schroeder, D.O.*

Books by Mary Summer Rain

Nonfiction
Spirit Song
Phoenix Rising
Dreamwalker
Phantoms Afoot
Earthway
Daybreak
Soul Sounds
Whispered Wisdom
Ancient Echoes
Bittersweet
Mary Summer Rain On Dreams
The Visitation
Millennium Memories
Fireside
Eclipse
The Singing Web
Beyond Earthway
Trined In Twilight
Pinecones
Love Never Sleeps

Fiction
The Seventh Mesa

Children's
Mountains, Meadows and Moonbeams
Star Babies

Books on Tape
Spirit Song
Phoenix Rising
Dreamwalker
Phantoms Afoot
The Visitation

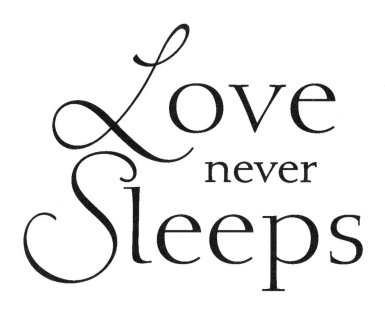

Love
never
Sleeps

MARY SUMMER RAIN

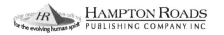

HAMPTON ROADS
PUBLISHING COMPANY, INC.

Cover design by Marjoram Productions
Cover photo by Mary Summer Rain

Hampton Roads Publishing Company, Inc.
1125 Stoney Ridge Road
Charlottesville, VA 22902

434-296-2772
fax: 434-296-5096
e-mail: hrpc@hrpub.com
www.hrpub.com

If you are unable to order this book from your local
bookseller, you may order directly from the publisher.
Call 1-800-766-8009, toll-free.

Library of Congress Catalog Card Number: 99-091421
ISBN: 1-57174-325-1
10 9 8 7 6 5 4 3 2 1
Printed on acid-free paper in Canada

For the Legacy of Knowledge and Understanding

that Mary Belle so graciously left to the world

through her encouragement for me to share

the story of her odyssey through Alzheimer's.

Table of Contents

Preface

This was not an easy book to write. In fact, for many reasons which will become evident to readers as they make their way through the book, it was probably the singularly most difficult volume of my entire list of nonfiction works to document, because of the uniquely specific type of societal experience it involved. When I'd finally finished the manuscript and several people at the publishing company had had a chance to peruse the material, I was surprised by some of the unexpected comments I received back in the way of general opinion and overall perception of its content. There appeared to be three major areas of concern about the book. Two of these ended up postponing its original publication schedule.

The first disturbing comment I heard regarding the manuscript dealt with the "tone" of it. Specifically, my tone. It was the opinion of some that, throughout the book, I sounded a bit, well . . . "hard" was the word that was used to describe it. When I heard this, rather than having hurt feelings or getting defensive, I experienced the opposite effect because it served to reinforce and doubly underscore my reasons for writing this book in the first place. That reasoning was the realization of the fact that most people out there just don't have a single clue as to everything that the Alzheimer's disease entails or, naturally, what an Alzheimer's caregiver goes through while providing daily care for a loved one afflicted with it.

Also, those individuals, both those at the publishing company and those who've been my faithful readers over the years, were accustomed to the very different type of material and style of writing contained in my previously published works that held much sensitivity toward nature and were generously spiced with lyrical, soul-stirring descriptions of the subtle "presence of the divine" in all things, and, most of all, how nature gives us unlimited examples of deep, yet simple, philosophical concepts that we can easily apply to our own daily lives as we interact with the various and myriad aspects of society—that is, *if* we would only stop to *see* and fully *appreciate* that enormously great potential for wisdom indwelling within all elements of life.

Therefore, both groups of people were used to my visually descriptive literary slant toward moonbeams, midnight mountain mists, and arching rainbows (nature's simple blessings to recognize and feel grateful for). And, obviously, this book isn't about any of those mentally pleasing imageries or matters. This book seemed to diverge straight into another realm of reality altogether: one of human disease. It was seen as a "medical" book.

So then, this last aspect also smoothly slid into what could be perceived as a subissue with the manuscript because, quite suddenly, I'd written something that was viewed as being allegedly "out of my genre"—*way* outside the realm of my genre, and that opinion seemed to cause some concerns related to marketability.

To be quite honest, on a personal level, I'd never previously felt that I'd been confined nor bound by any invisible chains connected to a definitively specific category of literary genre before this came up; after all, I'd written much poetry, two children's books, several straight-talking question-and-answer volumes, shared some personal life journals, and even published a novel. Though they all related in some way to philosophy (particularly spiritual philosophy), because the whole of my heretofore published writings had such a wide range that spanned so many types of diverse formats and subject matters associated with that elemental issue of spiritual philosophy, I didn't quite see how documenting the human behavioral performance of "unconditional love" and "unconditional goodness," as they're applied to the humanitarian task of being an Alzheimer's caregiver, could in any way be perceived as a great "divergence" from my long-established, core subject matter of spiritual behavior within society. The foundational concept of this book remains the same as that of most of my previous books. The underlying message is still related to the simple premise of applying spiritual philosophy to the everyday events in one's life through behavioral, hands-on application. I'd recognized a great societal need for a certain type of informational material, I'd personally gained the hands-on experience with it, so I wrote about it for the sole purpose of helping the many hundreds of people out there who are having to deal daily with the same type of situation. Whether one learns to utilize the behavioral applications of the spiritual philosophy of unconditional love and unconditional goodness through examples supplied by nature, or through the examples offered by various human diseases, it makes no difference. Whether the vector of the philosophical concept is found within nature or medicine is not germane. If it is, then someone's missing the whole point of this book. Yes. Granted, this is a medical book. Yet, it's also a book that clearly utilizes a medical venue to bring home a very simple and basic spiritual philosophy.

I believe those comments regarding my "tone" within this book came directly from a perspective based on expectation related to my former writings and that aforementioned "soft" type of material I'd presented in them. This book is not soft material. This book is a hard-hitting, honest look at Alzheimer's. It's a book that presents the disease's *clinical* behavioral characteristics in a *medically* symptomatic clear and straightforward manner that every individual can easily grasp and understand without filling it with a lot of high-minded medicalese language that goes over people's heads. To "soften" these detailed behavioral characteristics would be to seriously shortchange those who are seeking honest information about the disease and gravely compromise the integrity of the truth of its many characteristics. And, furthermore, to "soften" the types of physical and psychological burdens placed on the caregivers of those patients suffering from this disease would be doing a great disservice to those caregivers with respect to the wide array of emotions they can expect to feel while going through the experience of caring for a loved one with Alzheimer's in their home from onset to end stage.

It's not being emotionally "hard" when one is attempting to be completely honest in outlining all the clinical elements of a disease. And, I believe, that's possibly where the comments originated from. Perhaps, to some, it appeared that, while documenting the various behavioral characteristics of Alzheimer's, I was, in fact, "complaining" about them or not conveying enough emotional empathy for the patient while reporting on the myriad behavioral traits that are exhibited by the disease. Yet, clinical elements are clinical elements. The facts are the facts. This is not a sweetness 'n' light book describing leisurely ambles through sun-touched forests. Though it is a book written by a devoted naturalist whose heart and soul are deeply touched by every beautiful facet of nature, and who perceives deep philosophical lessons to be learned from each of them, the content of this one is about the *nature of a human disease* instead of the nature of Nature.

This is a book for *everyone* who wants to know the honest facts about dealing with a loved one with Alzheimer's. It's for *everyone*, everyone who wants the honest *truth* regarding what they can expect in the way of the disease's characteristic behavioral progression and the continual alterations that that behavior goes through as an afflicted loved one passes from one stage to the next, deepening one.

This book is for everyone who ever experienced the spear of fear that came with the passing thought that they may one day contract Alzheimer's themselves, or have to care one day for a parent who comes down with it. The facts may seem hard because, clinically, they are a hard reporting of the medical facts of the disease's behavioral characteristics and the deep impact they have on the at-home caregiver who lives with it twenty-four hours a day.

So this is a clinical book about two people's hour-by-hour job as at-home caregivers of a loved one with Alzheimer's. This is a clinical medical/psychological behavioral record of the disease's progression over a three-and-a-half-year period. If you're searching for the straightforward facts on this disease, this book's for you. If you're looking for a book that glosses over those facts with "soft" or sketchy, incomplete information that leaves the reader less informed than they should be about the disease after reading it, then look elsewhere. If you're looking for a tale about fairy rings and moonbeams, then this isn't the book for you. I'm not a "hard" person. Those who know me would scoff and shake their head at that description, yet a book detailing such a broad spectrum of the clinical behavioral elements of this specific disease is one that, inherently, *must* deal with the hard facts of it; otherwise, it gravely lacks integrity of purpose and fails to provide full disclosure. It must take a direct, head-on approach or it completely misses the whole point of even writing it.

The second major issue connected with the "original" manuscript was associated with the legality of honest reporting. By this I mean . . . those legal entanglements that can arise from being *too* honest.

When a family member is struck with a disease, familial complexities ensue. Because each family member is an individual possessing varied ideologies, opinions, life perspectives, and psychological compositions, each will exhibit separate responses to the fact that her/his loved one has contracted a terminal disease—especially if that loved one is a parent. Therefore, each family member will react in different ways. This is life. This is natural. However, from a literary point of view, reporting incidents of someone's ongoing negative behavior can sometimes present a legal problem for the author who documented it and for the publisher who allowed it to go public via the printed word. In the first draft of this book, without realizing it, I'd been far too thorough in detailing one of the participants' behavioral responses and, naturally, wishing to avoid the possibility of creating any legal issues from the material, I went back to page one and did a complete rewrite of the manuscript. This was one of the issues that eventually held up the book's originally scheduled publication date because I wasn't informed of this problem for quite some time.

The third issue that detained publication was the subject of "completion." Those in the publisher's editorial department felt that the book needed a conclusion whereby the caregivers could express their thoughts associated with the entire experience through the wisdom and after-knowledge of hindsight. I was informed about this at the same time as the legality issue and, to me, it meant that we were quite literally being asked to wait until the death of Sally's mother before the book would be brought to the "completion" that was desired by the editorial staff. To some of you reading this, that request may sound a bit "hard." Yet I understood the reasoning that was behind it. If this book was about caring for someone with a terminal disease from onset to endstage, then that endstage needed to be an inclusive element of the material. Hindsight, too, was an aspect that I hadn't originally thought to present in the material because my initial reason for doing the book was to clearly document all of the disease's varied behavioral characteristics and what the at-home caregiver can expect to experience while the patient is passing from one stage to the next. Yet much valuable information can be gleaned from the crystal clarity gained from that all-important hindsight perspective.

Clearly, regarding this disease and our experience with it, hindsight would ultimately answer the one glaring question many readers would naturally have—would we have done it all over again? Would we have placed our loved one in a nursing home? Hindsight would provide answers to questions regarding related treatments and the various methods of care we used at home. Was it worth all the emotional stress and loss of privacy and individual lifestyle freedom we experienced? Did the eventual daily sacrificing of self turn out to be a detrimental element to our overall psyche? Did we honestly feel we'd done our best—everything within our means—to give the optimum quality of care? What would we have done differently regarding the caregiving methodologies we utilized? How did we end up feeling after realizing that some of our thoughts during the process were not always what would be considered "spiritually admirable"? Was there anything we did to elicit "true" guilt as opposed to the naturally occurring "groundless" guilt often felt by such at-home caregivers? And lastly, how did we feel about the finality of it all?

So being asked to hold the publication of the book until the concluding event of the disease's endstage was reached and hindsight analysis of the whole situation was thoroughly examined was not a problem for me. I understood and respected the editorial staff's rationale of wanting to present a *completed* picture of what it's like caring for a loved one afflicted with Alzheimer's in one's home. Consequently, the manuscript was completely rewritten to accommodate the former legal issue by deleting the possibly offending statements, and, thereafter, the book was held in my computer as an "extended" ongoing work-in-progress. During that time I entered additional material as our patient's behavior continued to alter in a rapidly declining manner—always keeping the book updated and current in respect to the disease's end-stage progression. And when the time came, hindsight thoughts would be honestly examined and included, just as Mary Belle herself made us promise to do.

With the incidents of people contracting Alzheimer's disease on the rise, I would personally like to see more broad-spectrum media coverage of it. Not just news reports solely associated with the national and global numbers and percentages related to the disease's increasing rise in incidence, but perhaps more television movies made consisting of real-life, gut-honest portrayals depicting *factual* representations which give the general public a dose of reality that clearly reveals what it's *really* like for those family members giving daily care to an Alzheimer's-afflicted loved one in their home. The films and documentaries related to Alzheimer's that I've seen done for television viewing to date still haven't visually or explicitly reached down into the core of the patient's behavioral characteristics, but rather tended toward making subtly implied innuendoes to their nearly hidden reference, instead of graphically depicting them through visual dramatization. People's understanding of the full ramifications of the disease is foggy at best, and their intellectual comprehension of it remains elusive. Folks just have no idea. Through lack of straightforward information, they remain clueless.

This book was written for the prime purpose of bringing those mistaken ideas and missing clues to light. It was written to dispel the foggy misconceptions with a sweeping breeze of clarity and to transform the elusiveness of intellectual perception into one of sharp definition.

Introduction

In July of 1996, my friend Sally and I jointly bought a modest two-bedroom cedar cabin overlooking a secluded valley on ten acres high up in the Colorado Rocky Mountains. The structure had never been lived in due to the fact that the initial construction on it began in 1983, and had since been the recreational, weekend building project of two, not-so-handy former owners. Consequently, the dwelling boasted of plywood floors, Sheetrock walls, gaping electrical outlets, missing bathroom plumbing, and no electricity save that provided by an old hospital generator that leaked motor oil like a torn, wire sieve and guzzled propane like a fuel-starved monster.

These questionable attributes didn't deter us, though, because the dwelling was pleasingly situated at the end of a quarter-mile-long, winding drive through a towering forest of fragrant pine, blue spruce, and thick aspen stands. The spectacular beauty and tranquility of the pastoral setting created a touchable presence that the heart and soul couldn't ignore. After standing on the covered front porch and casting my gaze out over the peaceful valley below, I knew with every fiber of my being that this was "the" place. This was the place that would provide me with the therapeutic solitude and serenity that I needed after recently traveling over some very rough life roads.

And so we bought the place and immediately plunged into long days and nights of doing the finishing work ourselves. We worked on getting carpet down, installing bathroom sinks, tubs, and showers, finishing the electrical work, building a large fenced-in dog yard (with a cover of chicken wire to keep the resident hawks and owls from swooping down and snapping up our tiny Yorkies for a snack), building two separate sets of railroad tie stairs and staining, installing, and varnishing knotty pine, tongue-in-groove paneling to cover the interior walls. We managed to fully complete the work on the ground floor, the upstairs bath, and my bedroom before we ran out of money (and space on our combined credit cards) to finish paneling Sally's bedroom and the stairwell.

Not being connected to the power grid didn't faze us in the least because we actually liked the simple living it afforded us. We liked it a lot because there was a certain sense of independence and self-sufficiency associated with being off the grid system that everyone else depended so heavily on. Yet, just out of curiosity and for our own information, we checked out what the change-over would cost to have it brought in. Well! Such a deal! We could have it brought underground to our cabin for a mere $27,000—the full amount paid up front! No installment payments accepted. Whew! That information was a real shocker and we definitely had to catch our breaths after hearing that little bit of news. We each quickly thanked our lucky stars that we really didn't *want* to be connected and had absolutely, positively *no* plans for ever doing so! The way we saw it, why on earth *would* we when we were so perfectly content with just the way things were?

Happily we ditched the old, inefficient generator by selling it to a generator repair shop that wanted it for spare parts. We made a whopping $100 on the deal and, after some finagling, we managed to come up with the cash for a small Wacker gasoline generator. After installing the new one in a more convenient place beneath the front porch (one we could walk under), Sally wired it into the electrical circuit box and we were satisfied that we not only had our own power source, but we were also prepared to carry on life-as-usual in the face of any future emergency. It was a good little generator that adequately handled our basic necessities and, on the average, we ran it fourteen hours a day, seven days a week.

Living off the grid was a whole new world to get used to, though. The situation demands many lifestyle changes. Most of the time the refrigerator ran on brown-out power and was completely off all night long when we shut down the generator upon retiring. From various interesting experiences (some funny and some not so hilarious) we quickly learned which appliances pulled too much power to use. We couldn't use a microwave, an electric coffee pot (forget the espresso and Sally's bread maker), or any kitchen or bathroom electrical appliance. After many experimental starts and stops of trial and error, we learned the ins and outs of living with a generator as our sole source of electrical power. We discovered that we could only run the vacuum or iron when the water pump and hot water tank weren't running. We could have television (snowy with rooftop antenna) only when one of us wasn't taking a shower—the shower kicked on the hot water tank and well pump. I blew the Canon copy machine when I first tried to use it, so that piece of office equipment was quickly relegated to the basement. I could efficiently operate my IBM typewriter, but we couldn't have an answering machine on the phone or even have a portable unit because we didn't have the all-night power to hold a charge on either piece of equipment.

We adjusted. We adjusted just fine. Life was good and would've been perfect if it hadn't been for the singular exception of the small irritation of the generator noise which drowned out the birdsong, wind through the pines, and coyote calls. But we'd take care of that by turning off the generator for a couple of afternoon hours, just so we could enjoy the sounds of wind and wildlife and soak up nature's peaceful aura around our little dwelling.

We still had endless projects lined up, but those were merely viewed as anticipated work providing a healthy means of good physical exercise, like getting out in the woods with the chainsaw to turn the deadfall and diseased aspen trees into cords of winter firewood and to collect boxes of kindling.

Sally was kept busy with construction labors from daybreak to twilight, while I, being the writer, divided my time between routine housework, giving her a hand with the more difficult tasks, and doing research to keep my writing projects up. There was always something to do. There was always a long string of construction or repair jobs waiting in line behind the one we were currently working on. Boredom wasn't something we were familiar with. When it came time to turn the generator off at night and take our flashlights up to our respective rooms, we were tired and could expect to sleep the kind of sound slumber that comes from a hard day's work. Daybreak would arrive soon enough to greet us with another full measure of healthy and emotionally fulfilling activities.

Life continued on this way, working on never-ending cabin projects and writing books until, fifteen months later, something unexpected happened that completely altered our daily routine. Sally suddenly was presented with the urgent need to bring her elderly mother, Mary Belle, out here to live with us and, my friend having completely given up her room for her mother's sole use, resigned herself to storing all of her own personal items in boxes in the basement and to sleeping down on the living room love seat.

Initially, we thought we were simply dealing with her mother's purely physical health problems, but we soon discovered that the condition was far more complex and far-reaching. It was also Alzheimer's.

After this was clearly evident, even before she was professionally diagnosed, we bought dozens of books on the subject and found a glaring void in the type of information available to the general public. Most of the volumes were either written by doctors or by family members who had their Alzheimer's-afflicted loved ones ensconced in nursing homes. Of the many books we researched, none were actually written by adult children who were personally caring for a parent or other related loved one *in their own home*. This specific scenario is a completely different circumstance that presents a more sophisticated set of complex emotional entanglements for the caregiver. It's one thing to visit a parent with Alzheimer's a couple times a week in a nursing home, but it becomes a whole different experience to have to continually deal with it twenty-four hours a day in your own home. And this situation has proven, beyond any shadow of a doubt, that . . . love never sleeps.

After having Mary Belle here for a few months, it became crystal clear that we no longer had the luxury of our chosen option to stay off the power grid as we'd planned. Due to the generator being off all night we had no power to the water well pump or lights during that time and she couldn't remember to refrain from flushing toilets or trying to run water. She'd also forget that she needed to use her bedside flashlight if she needed to get out of bed. Without light she began making her soundless way downstairs to roam about the dark house and, eventually, wander out the back door, through the garden gate, and into the even darker woods (we've had bears and coyotes come up to the house even during the daylight hours). The nighttime darkness of the house proved to be too unsafe for this frail, elderly woman. We had no choice but to bite the proverbial bullet. We again contacted the electric company, this time for the purpose of contracting for a power installation. We were not at all happy, but there was no way around it if we wanted to provide a safer environment for Sally's mother by lessening the hazards that the lack of electricity presented during the night.

This book, on the whole, is written by myself as an at-home caregiver unrelated to the patient. As this unrelated individual, I'm in the convenient position of being once removed from the familial emotional entanglements of the situation and can stand back to objectively observe the interaction of family members, not only the obvious relationship between Sally and her mother, but also the psychological machinations of her two adult siblings and their own completely different sets of behavioral reactions to having a parent with Alzheimer's.

In my in-depth research into (and invaluable firsthand experience with) this specific dementia disease, I've found that the various individualized, psychological elements of the adult children play a monumental role that weaves a tightly interrelated web of complexities into the situation. This aspect is a major, recognized factor associated with Alzheimer's that is not prevalently evident in other types of parent-related diseases or illnesses.

Having now had over three and a half years' worth of twenty-four-hours-a-day experience with this disease, I've also come to recognize this unique situation as presenting a viable and invaluable opportunity to practice the spiritual philosophy of unconditional goodness and acceptance. This Alzheimer's condition and the situation of relatives and caregivers being directly involved with it makes for the quintessential circumstance to turn one's spiritual *beliefs* into those of personally applied corporeal acts of spiritual *works* in the world—to manifest their spiritual goodness in a real hands-on manner by way of positive behavioral responses—and provides the precious opportunity to spiritually grow through the attainment of greater depths of matured wisdom.

It is for this reason that Sally and I have collaborated on writing this book. We've written it not only to help the general public broaden their personal understanding and knowledge of this disease and to assist the at-home caregivers with proven methods of coping with it, but to also exemplify how this singular situation presents itself as being a wonderful opportunity for the twenty-four-hour caregiver to gain the grace of patience, the strength of acceptance, and the recognition of the myriad ways it offers the individual the chance to develop and attain a greater measure of wisdom through the incredible power of love.

Due to the fact that only Sally knows the complete details of her own mother's history, she has written the first section, which is highly important from the standpoint of the reader gaining a clear understanding of how and why her mother came to be here with us. The rest of the material has been written by myself, after much discussion between Sally and me, and is filled with many actual examples of the typical types of challenging behavior the caregiver is presented with and "expected" to handle with grace on a daily basis. Together, we offer this volume as an invaluable aid for all at-home caregivers in their ongoing efforts to genuinely feel and express continued love for their parents or loved ones in the face of seemingly insurmountable odds. The multitude of varying elements associated with this particular disease can oftentimes make this seem like an ostensibly impossible goal to achieve. I've seen this. I know this to be true. It's an extremely difficult situation. Love sometimes wants to sleep, to take a short catnap for emotional respite, but it can't; it can't, because it may very well never wake up again. And that's why we've written this book.

I. Some Background History
by Sally

Some Background History

It was the second week of October in 1997, and, for my money, it was the most magical time of year in the high Rocky Mountains. The lapis depths of the clear autumn sky made a brilliant backdrop when looking up through the golden undersides of the aspen leaves that shimmered and quaked in the light breeze.

I was out in the woods and had three-fourths of the upcoming winter's cordwood cut. There was something special about being out in the fragrant air of the autumn forest that made me feel especially healthy and wonderfully invigorated. The physical exercise in the crisp atmosphere combined with the soul's solitary communion with nature and, as a result, I felt gifted with a heightened feeling of overall exhilaration. It was a feeling of total well-being. It was good, so good. Life was good.

I loaded the last of the day's labors into the bed of the battered pickup and headed back down the winding driveway toward home to unload and stack it. After backing the truck behind the cabin, I started tossing the cut logs onto the ground. My friend Mary came out of the cabin to help stack. She had barely begun the process when she dashed back into the house to answer the phone. Quickly returning to the door, she called out that my sister, Judy, needed to speak to me.

The message wasn't encouraging. The previous night, Judy had experienced an emergency with our mother, Mary Belle. She'd had to call an ambulance, and my mother was currently in the hospital. Judy repeatedly assured me that Mom seemed to be okay now, and, since the doctors didn't find anything major wrong, she probably wouldn't be in the hospital for long. The physicians' initial assessment was that perhaps Mom had simply forgotten to take her high blood pressure medication. After I immediately responded to this news by telling Judy that I was going to pack a bag and be there the following day, she too quickly said that I didn't need to come. Her response struck me as being more than a little odd, because I certainly wanted to be there with my mother in her time of need.

Judy and my mother both lived in Overland Park, Kansas, not too far from each other. That's where I'd been living before moving out to Colorado three years earlier. Previously, Mary Belle and I had shared a beautiful piece of residential property with nearly a half-acre of lawn. She resided in the primary house while I lived in a small guest house set toward the back of the yard. With this arrangement, I was easily able to take care of mother's outside work, do house repairs, take her places and, generally, keep watch over her when I wasn't at work. When personal circumstances in my life made it necessary for me to move out of state, we sold the high-maintenance property and bought her a very nice ground floor, two-bedroom townhouse that was more suitable and convenient for her to take care of, and my sister took over the responsibility of keeping a close eye on her. As far as I knew, this arrangement was working out well and mother had been having no problems; in fact, she seemed quite content with the situation. When I called her, several times a week routinely since moving away, she'd always conveyed a light-hearted attitude and never complained of anything ever being amiss in her life.

After I got off the phone with Judy, I called the hospital and was able to talk directly to Mom. She was very vague about the specifics of her own current physical condition. I had the distinct sense that she wasn't quite sure how she was or what was really going on. Formerly, Judy had told me that she was going to go over to the hospital to check on Mom that evening, so I decided that it'd be best if I waited and called Judy after she could supply more complete information about our mother's condition. This subsequent call to her yielded no new knowledge, though. Other than the fact that the medical team was having trouble getting Mom's medication regulated, I could learn nothing new. I was very concerned and this informational void wasn't acceptable to me. It was extremely frustrating being so far away. I called Mary Belle again and she said she wanted me there with her. Her trembling voice sounded desperately pleading and pulled at my heartstrings.

My friend and I sat down and fully discussed the situation as it wasn't exactly the best time, weatherwise, to leave Colorado. I was in the middle of cutting the winter's supply of firewood and, at our mountain elevation of nearly *9900* feet, it wouldn't be a bit unusual to wake up one of these mornings to a couple of feet of new-fallen snow. Yet, both Mary and I felt that I should go and see if I could be of some help to my mother. I packed a bag, attended to a few essential things around the house like making sure there was enough gasoline and oil in storage for the generator, and took off early the following morning for Kansas.

The drive took me twelve hours and I went directly to the hospital upon arriving in town at 7 P.M. that evening. Mary Belle's room was a private one in the cardiac unit of Shawnee Mission Hospital. What I walked in on appalled me. I couldn't believe my eyes. My mother was tied to her bed in a Velcro restraint contraption. I hadn't been informed of this very unusual aspect of my mother's situation. Nobody was currently in the room with her and it took her a few moments to recognize who I was. As soon as she did, she started to literally beg me to take her home, to get her out of this place. *Now!*

I managed to calm her down somewhat and attempted to shift her mind from the subject before leaving her in search of someone who could tell me why the hell my mother was tied to her bed.

Exiting the room, I strode down the hall to the nurses' station and found an appropriate-looking woman who I thought might be able to enlighten me. As calmly as I could, I identified myself as Mary Belle's daughter, and asked my burning question. The woman looked at me sideways while picking up my mother's chart, and mumbling something about her "having been seriously disoriented." What that precisely meant, I didn't know and this woman obviously did not want to commit herself to making a full-blown, explanatory statement so she opted to inform me that, "you can catch your mother's doctor if you're here first thing in the morning."

"First thing in the *morning?*" I impatiently shot back in a voice dripping with disdain. "Excuse me, but my mother is tied to her bed!" Respectfully keeping the expletives to myself, I turned away from the desk and went back into mother's room where I immediately got on the phone with my sister. I figured that surely Judy would know what was going on, and, at the same time, wondered where she was. It was in the middle of prime time visiting hours at the hospital and I'd expected to see her there. When the phone was answered at my sister's house, it was the voice of one of my nephews that I heard. He said that his Mom was out making her Avon deliveries but he thought she was going to stop by the hospital when she was finished. We ended the conversation, and I felt alone and extremely frustrated over the entire situation.

So now what?

Hurry up and wait. That's the first rule of our medical system, is it not? So I started up a conversation with Mom in an effort to pass the time. She desperately wanted to go back home and, through various means, also let me know that she perceived my arrival as being her only ticket out.

At around 8:30 P.M. Judy came through the door and, by the expression on her face, I could see that she was literally shocked to see me, as I'd come into town without letting anyone know I'd arrived. She appeared outwardly disconcerted to realize that I'd actually made the drive. She immediately began telling me that I hadn't really needed to make the trip and be there because Mom had been doing pretty good.

"Judy," I politely said behind a tightly clenched jaw, "let's take a walk. We need to talk."

Once outside the room she started to explain that, after the procedures in the emergency room, Mom had become disoriented and physically combative with the medical personnel. She went on to explain that the doctors were telling her that it wasn't unusual for a person of Mom's age (79) to be disoriented for a few days after such an episode and that they fully expected her to snap out of it. They had started her on some medication to help and wanted to continue monitoring her for a few more days.

I was not only physically exhausted from the long drive but had been met with what appeared to me to be some very contradictory and confusing events that needed to be sorted out. Clearly, Judy had not fully disclosed the extent of my mother's situation over the phone, and I wondered why. Deciding that my wisest next move was to get some rest and then talk to the doctor myself in the morning, I got Mom's house keys from Judy and left for the evening after telling Mom goodnight and informing her that I was going to head over to her house to take care of her schnauzer, Molly. This appeared to appease her for the moment, as she was thoroughly devoted to that dog. I assured her that I would be back to see her first thing in the morning and that we'd get some of this mess straightened out for her—or so I thought. Little did I realize that the surprises were just beginning.

Relieved to reach the townhouse for some much-needed peace and quiet, I opened the door and flipped on the light.

Another surprise.

I couldn't believe my eyes.

The deplorable condition of the place was shocking. Mom had always been an impeccable housekeeper, having specific household chores for each day of the week. I saw no evidence of this. Instead, I was confronted with clutter everywhere I looked. Stacks of envelopes with rubber bands wrapped around them lined the tops of the furniture eight to ten inches deep. Dirty dishes were all over the kitchen. The light beige carpet had become brown through the center walkways. The bathroom was in desperate need of a thorough cleaning. And her bedroom was in disarray from the visit of the ambulance crew a couple of nights earlier.

After a quick assessment of the place, I retrieved my bag from the car and tossed it into the guest room. I hadn't had anything to eat so I checked the fridge. Big mistake. I couldn't believe what I was looking at. Mary Belle had only been in the hospital for a couple of days, yet everything—and I mean everything—from the lettuce to the lunch meat was moldy and nasty. It was obvious that the food had been sitting like this for many days, not just a couple. This was not at all like her.

Incredulous, I just shut the door, got a cup out of the cupboard, and made myself instant coffee with hot tap water. The increasingly incongruous elements of the situation I was seeing were not adding up. They were mystifying. Something about my mother's life appeared to be very much amiss.

Before I could think any more about these odd events, I sat down in the dining room and placed a long-overdue call to my friend back home. I couldn't put off that call any longer, because it was already after midnight in Colorado and I knew that Mary would be anxiously waiting to hear that I'd arrived safely and also how my mother was faring.

She answered after two rings and it was good to hear her voice. She said that she and the dogs were all doing just fine, and then she sympathetically listened to what I had to say about my unusual day. As soon as we hung up I went into the bathroom and began cleaning. I cleaned until around 3 A.M. and then, exhausted, dropped onto the top of the bed.

The alarm clock was screaming at 6 A.M. and, in a mental haze, I pulled off the clothes I'd fallen asleep in and made my foggy way to the shower. I managed to make it to the hospital by seven and was greatly relieved to find out that the doctor hadn't yet been in.

Mary Belle was still restrained in her bed and had a patient "sitter" in a chair beside her. The young man was glad to see me and hear that I would be there all day. He promptly left to attend to other duties.

I didn't have to wait long for Dr. Thompson to enter the room. He briefly checked out his patient and then started out the door. I followed close on his heels. He told me that my mother had been admitted with rapid atrial fibrillation and prolonged chest pain. He added that her cardiac enzymes were borderline positive and so they'd done a cardiac catheterization which showed moderate three-vessel coronary artery disease. Apparently, when she had come to the emergency room, she'd been fairly lucid and had been able to give the doctors a general medical history of herself. I asked him about the extreme mental confusion that she was exhibiting and he reiterated what my sister had said about age and the expected improvement. I then asked him if the restraints could be taken off of her while I was there to watch over her and he readily agreed. I went back into the room and, in half an hour, a nurse came to remove the straps around her wrists. Mom seemed greatly appeased by this new freedom and acted both happy and relieved to know that I was there with her. Together we passed the morning watching the game shows on her TV.

At lunch time they brought her some hospital food and she quickly turned her nose up. She needed to eat well to regain her strength, so I went over to the cafeteria and brought back something that I thought would be more appetizing to her. It was. She appeared to be extremely tired, and I knew from past experience that every time the doctors changed her medication, it took her some days of adjustment for her system to get itself regulated to it.

After she'd eaten, she soundly slept for the rest of the afternoon. She seemed to be so exhausted that it was as though she hadn't slept in days. Today was the 13th of October and the fall colors were just starting to appear in Kansas City. This Midwestern flora, so different from the western mountains' foliage shapes and colors I'd become used to, brought a sense of awe of the wide variety of natural beauty existing in all of creation. The window of Mother's room faced southwest and the golden orb of the sun was just beginning to lower along the horizon as they brought in her dinner tray. I released a heavy sigh as I turned my back on the retiring sun and mentally returned to the reality of the hospital room.

The nurse woke my mother and sat her up in the bed before she left to deliver another patient's meal. I watched as Mom made a valiant effort to eat; she poked her fork around the tray but didn't get too much eaten. She asked me to get rid of the tray, so I took it into the hall and set it on the cart. Her phone rang then. It was Mom's friends, Kathryn and Louise, from church. They said they were on their way over to see her and I felt encouraged that her friends were coming by to visit. She needed cheering and I hoped that seeing her longtime friends would be just the good medicine to do the trick.

Kathryn had been in a bad traffic accident several years back and now used a wheelchair much of the time. I told them I would meet them at the hospital entrance. After telling the nurses that I was going downstairs to meet someone, I roamed the halls until I found an extra wheelchair, appropriated it for Kathryn, and headed for the front door. The timing was perfect. They pulled up just as I got to the door. Kathryn climbed into the wheelchair and Louise took off to park the car.

As I wheeled her through the doors and into the lobby, Kathryn said with great disdain in her voice, "Why haven't you gotten here sooner? Your mother needs some help?"

I didn't know how to respond to that, because, as far as I knew, Mom had been getting along just fine, and Judy had always assured me that she'd been taking care of her. Kathryn's statement baffled me. What the hell did she mean by that? Just then Louise came through the door and the three of us headed up to Mary Belle's room before I had a chance to question Kathryn further. Mom was thrilled to see them, and, wanting to give them some privacy together, I went back downstairs in search of some sugar-free candy in the gift shop, because Kathryn is diabetic.

After browsing around for about half an hour to kill some time, I returned to Mom's room with my hands full of goodies and some magazines for her to pass the time looking through. Her company stayed a while longer and shared light conversation about church folks and current social activities. Finally they asked me if I would walk them out and help get Kathryn back into the car. As we made our way to the parking lot I told them what the doctor had said that morning and what shocking conditions I'd found both at the hospital and in the townhouse when I'd arrived. We made plans to talk later when we all had more time.

It was getting late and I hadn't seen my sister all day. The nurses were acting like it was time for me to leave. I said my goodnights to Mom, kissed her, and left with the excuse that I needed to attend to her dog, promising to be back first thing in the morning. She didn't want me to go, but resigned herself to the parting.

On the way to the townhouse, I stopped by Judy's house to pick up Mom's dog and greet my niece and three nephews. Only the kids and their dad were home. My sister was out delivering her Avon orders. I visited with the family until Judy finally arrived home. Not wishing to immediately put her on the defensive, I decided not to say anything about her absence from the hospital all day, but did ask about the deplorable condition of Mom's townhouse. The answers were not satisfactory to me. I was so tired after having gotten only three hours' sleep the night before that I cut right to the chase and tried to pin her down about when she would be at the hospital the following day. I received no firm reply. Exasperated, I took the dog and left, stopping at Burger King on the way home to get Molly and myself a quick meal.

Once back at the townhouse, I again placed a call to Mary to check in and keep her informed of the ongoing situation as it was unfolding. We were both anxious for me to be able to return home and resume my current woodcutting project before the snow flew. I had also taken our only semi-reliable vehicle, which left her with no way to leave the cabin. One of our friends had lent her a vehicle to use in my absence, but it leaked brake fluid and she told me that, on one of her excursions into town to get the mail, the brakes got mushy on her while she was descending down a hairpin curve, and, by the time she left town to make the ascent up the mountain, the brakes were going all the way down to the floor. She'd eased it home safely, yet couldn't use it anymore. Her son-in-law took her to the gas station a couple of times to refill the generator gas cans, and friends were bringing her the mail and anything else she needed while I was away. My heart sank when she told me about her close call with the brakes, and I was relieved to hear that all ended well with that potentially dangerous event. After the call, I took Molly for a walk and then watched television for mental diversion until I finally fell asleep in the chair.

The following morning I was at the hospital by 7 A.M. and, to my great disappointment, once more found my mother tied down with restraints. The fellow sitting in the room with her told me that she'd had a rough night, and then he left to get himself a cup of coffee. I went up to my mother and smoothed back her disheveled hair. She looked up at me with pleading eyes and told me that she desperately needed to use the restroom. I undid the wrist restraints, helped her into the bathroom and shut the door behind her while I respectfully waited outside. I was leaning against the hallway door when my mother suddenly exited the bathroom without a stitch of clothing on and defiantly announced, "I'm getting out of here!"

Wide-eyed and aghast, I sputtered, "Mom! You can't go out there like that! You aren't dressed!"

She didn't say a thing. Instead of making any verbal response or showing any sign of concern that she was as naked as a newborn babe, she just began trying to physically push past me. When she realized that I wasn't going to budge from the doorway, she took one calculated step back and began slapping my face; first with one hand, then with the other. I was in such disbelief and utter shock that I didn't even attempt to defend myself. Instead, I found that I was just counting the blows. Finally, after the tenth or eleventh slap, I came to my senses. I grabbed both of her wrists and wrestled her back to the bed where I could reach the call button. When the nurse arrived, I asked for help dressing my mother without "telling" on her about the slapping incident because, to me, that somehow felt like a very dishonorable thing for a daughter to do. Noticing that the patient was agitated after being dressed in a gown and robe, the nurse suggested that I walk her around the hallways to give her some exercise.

My mother heard this.

Out the door she flew.

The nurse and I were hot on her heels.

She headed straight for the Exit sign. Well, the door led to a stairwell and it took both the nurse and me to pry Mom's hands off the door handle. She'd had her fingers around it like a vise. When she was finally convinced that she wasn't getting any access to that exit, she again took off down the hall, this time entering the ICU. Finding an empty room, she immediately entered and sat down. It seemed that she thought that we'd just go away if she sat there long enough.

In the meantime, the nurse and I stood outside the room talking about the situation and, while we were discussing this, we noticed Mary Belle trying to sneak behind us and around the unit toward another door. We followed at a distance, yet I was actually jogging to keep up with her fast pace.

We watched Mom try to open every door and, eventually, every window she came to. The fact that she actually tried to open windows made my heart sink. Would she actually go out of a window? Would she really consider jumping? I shuddered at the thought but didn't have time to dwell on it.

The nurse and I were finally successful in corralling mother back into her room where another nurse met up with us to assist us in getting her back into bed. Mom sat down on the edge of the bed and sighed. When I reached down to take off her slippers, she suddenly picked up the telephone off the nightstand and slammed it down on my head. Pausing to clear the stars from my vision, I stood, and the nurses guided me from the room. They seemed to believe that their patient's agitation was directed at me for some unknown reason and wanted to get her back into the restraints. I was beginning to think that, if this uncharacteristic behavior of aggression continued, they were going to kick her out of the hospital. My former attitude about the restraints was also beginning to change. One of the nurses returned with some medication, and the other one told me that she'd have a doctor stop by as soon as he was free. Shortly afterward, he entered the room and sat with Mom a bit before he then rose to leave, saying that he'd return with his written assessment.

Mother acted as though nothing out of the ordinary had just happened. She seemed perfectly okay with the idea of me leaving the room for awhile. I took advantage of her amenable attitude and left to get myself some coffee and much-needed space to think over the recent events that'd left my mind reeling.

Not wanting to miss the doctor, I had my coffee and decided to leave the more in-depth thinking for later. I went straight back to the room. As it turned out, I didn't need to rush back so soon because it was a few hours later when he showed up. He was a small, dark man with kind, compassionate eyes. His report reads as follows:

Mary Belle is a 79-year-old patient who was admitted to the cardiology unit through the Emergency Room, referred because of chest pain. She was diagnosed with atrial flutter.

The patient is unable to give a good history at this point. Much of the information is obtained from the patient's daughter, who lives in Colorado and who was visiting at the time of consultation, as well as discussions with the nursing staff. It appears that Mary Belle had been functioning fairly independently until very recently, when she was admitted to the hospital for chest pain, palpitations, and had been undergoing some tests. Over the past couple of days, staff and daughter report that patient had become increasingly confused, not sleeping well at night, racing thoughts, some disorientation, confusion, and, within the past several hours, had become kind of agitated, combative, and even had struck her daughter with the telephone. As per family, this type of behavior was very unusual for the patient.

No prior psychiatric history. No prior history of any alcohol or drug abuse type of problems.

The patient lives independently. She has two daughters and a son. One daughter lives in Kansas City. Family is supportive.

PAST MEDICAL HISTORY: Significant for history of angina, hypertension, carotid endarterectomy several years ago. The patient had cerebrovascular accident with some speech impediment within the past several years.

CURRENT MEDICATIONS: Norvasc 5mg a day, Lanoxin 0.125mg q.o.d., Metoprolol 50mg b.i.d., Nitro-Dur patch, Temazepam 15mg at h.s. p.r.n., Haldol p.r.n. 0.5 to 1mg.

MENTAL STATUS EXAMINATION: Reveals a 79-year-old, white female who is resting in bed. She is not fully alert with moderate degree of confusion. She is disoriented to time and place. Her concentration and attention span appear impaired. She is unable to recall recent and past events. Intelligence, as evidenced by vocabulary, appears to be average. She denies any thoughts of harm to self or others. The patient is relatively calm at this time and attempts to cooperate with interview. The patient is unable to cooperate fully with mini-mental status exam but significant deficits are noted. Motor activity is mildly increased.

IMPRESSION:
AXIS I: Delirium, not otherwise specified.
AXIS II: No disorder.
AXIS III: Angina.
       Hypertension.
       History of carotid endarterectomy.
       Cerebrovascular accident.
AXIS IV: Moderate degree of stressors, health problems.
AXIS V: Current global assessment of function 35 to 40, highest in the past year 65 to 70.

RECOMMENDATIONS:
1. Haldol 0.5 mg q. 6 to 8 hours p.r.n. for agitation.
2. Trazodone 25 mg h.s. for insomnia.

3. MRI of head.
4. Social assessment to look at the living situation and placement alternative.

Thank you for the opportunity to assist in care of this patient. Will follow as needed. May want to consider transfer to psychiatric unit after medical stabilization for further evaluation and management.

The order for the MRI was at my insistence. There had to be an explanation for my mother's oddly uncharacteristic combative behavior and I wanted any and all physiological causes checked out. Perhaps she had suffered another stroke. I knew Mom had experienced a couple of small stroke events last spring and had undergone some subsequent speech therapy throughout the following summer months. She also had been doing volunteer work at another hospital, going to church every Sunday, driving her car wherever she needed to go, playing Bingo, and, otherwise, as far as I knew, living a fairly normal and independently self-sufficient life for someone her age. Having always been very close to my family, I'd called Mom several times a week to check up on her and mostly just to chat. I had also been calling my sister more often to get her continuing assessment of Mom and her situation. I was always informed that "everything was just fine with Mom." Now I was beginning to wonder if my sister and I had very opposing definitions of "fine."

As you may have noted while reading the doctor's official report, I have a brother. Tony lives in North Carolina and calls his mother at least once a week. Throughout my visit back to Kansas I had been keeping in close touch with him by phone, usually on the pay phone in the hall of the hospital. It was easier to catch him at his office, and, because of the time differential, by the time I left the hospital each evening and got to Mom's townhouse, he was already in bed for the night.

17

Soon after the doctor gave his report, he left the room. Shortly afterward, a nurse came in to inform me that they'd be taking Mom down for the MRI in a few minutes. She made it a point to specifically ask me if I would personally accompany Mom, because they were naturally concerned that she'd become agitated again during the procedure. In addition, she asked me to keep a close eye on Mother and to please not leave her *while the procedure was taking place.* Not that I would've anyway, but I reassured her that I would, indeed, stay close by.

I wondered where my sister was. I'd made several calls asking her to be there for the MRI, so she could personally hear what the doctor had to say about the results and, particularly, to be there with me to give our mother joint moral support and comfort. My thoughts on this were interrupted when the transport attendant came to take Mom downstairs to the imaging room. It was time for the MRI.

If you've never had the MRI test, for some people, it can be a fairly daunting procedure to experience. You're taken into a room full of space age-looking equipment and you lie down on a hard, cold surface. They strapped Mom down and left her in the room alone, shutting the heavy metal door behind them. Next, the operator sat down at a vast array of dials, buttons, computer screens—you get the idea—and he started it up while observing her through a window. The table began to move and she entered a cocoon-like machine where she was inundated, for a time, with booming noises. Because the nurse had been so adamant about me keeping a close eye on my mother, I stood right there watching her through the window, half anticipating her to panic at any moment. I hadn't said a word to the technician fellow operating the machine, but, somehow, my presence appeared to really annoy him, and he told me to go sit in the waiting room.

"Excuse me," I responded, "but that is my mother in there, and just who do you think is paying for you to run this test?" I was livid as I told him what the nurse had repeatedly stressed to me about staying close to my mother during the procedure.

He was insistent.

I'd been standing on the other side of a four-foot counter from him and had specific instructions to keep a close eye on my mother. Since the tech was informed of that and remained unfazed, my first thought was that the procedure wasn't evincing good news and that, perhaps, he didn't want me to see the results.

After he'd finished and Mary Belle was brought out, I began to imagine all sorts of horrid possibilities. I knew I wouldn't get any kind of adequate answer until the doctor had looked at the test results and also had the time and inclination to share them. As may be becoming more and more apparent, I personally don't think much of hospitals.

In 1972, my father had an epileptic-like seizure during our family's Thanksgiving dinner. We immediately called 911 and had him rushed to St. Luke's Hospital, where they ran a variety of tests and found absolutely nothing in the way of a physiological cause. Then, on the following New Year's Day, he had another attack, and back we went. My mother, brother, sister, and I were in the hospital's very public and crowded waiting room filled with complete strangers when the doctor strode right up to my mother and, without a pause or hesitation or any quiet note of empathy in his tone, flatly said, "Rudy has a malignant tumor the size of a baseball in his brain and will only live about three months." The doctor then coldly announced that they were admitting him. The "professional" then turned his back to us and briskly walked away.

Dad was 56, very active, and always exceptionally healthy. This was indeed a low blow that struck out from some very black hole. He lived for a year and a half after that, enduring the rigors of brain surgery, some of the very first experimental chemotherapy treatments, which made him so sick he would spend entire days with his head over the toilet. The doctors wanted us to admit him to a nursing home, but he wanted to be in his own home, so that's exactly where we brought him.

One of my more memorable experiences throughout it all was going into his room and finding him with a 104-degree temperature. We rushed him to the hospital again and anxiously stood beside his bed while listening to a neurosurgeon order a spinal tap to discover the source of the infection. On dad's left forearm there was a large, swollen, red area about four inches in diameter with evident infection in the center. So, being bold and outspoken for my years, I'd said to this neurosurgeon, "That looks like a spider bite to me. Could that be the cause?"

It was.

The doctor had made the false assumption that the skin redness was merely a bedsore and hadn't even examined it closer, but was more than eager to make my already tortured father endure yet another painful procedure without, as far as I was concerned, looking for the obvious. At that point in my life I made up my mind to always make my own final medical decisions. M.D.s or not, common sense and an awareness of the obvious had to play a part in the overall assessment of a diagnosis.

This was just one of many such experiences.

Another was entering my father's hospital room more than once and finding him feeling physically miserable and emotionally humiliated, as he was left lying in his own bodily waste. After that happened, he was never left alone again as either Mom or I was always there at his side to make sure he was comfortable and "clean."

Rudy passed away at home, as he wanted to, with his family all around him. He was 58 years of age. The death of a loved one, even if it's been imminent and expected, can be a traumatic emotional blow that affects those left behind in a variety of ways. Everyone deals with death differently, and,

I believe, a part of my mother also died that hot, summer night because, to this day, I wonder if it wasn't the spark that set her course down the road leading to who she is today. She was never quite the same after that.

As they carried my father's body out the front door of the house and put him into the awaiting hearse, I couldn't determine if it was a wail or a scream, but my mother made a chilling sound that still haunts me to this day. The closest I've ever heard to it is the scream of an injured rabbit.

Primal and feral.

Heartrending.

Truly bone-chilling.

With my mother's MRI completed, the attendant arrived to transport her back up to her room. Soon after we returned, a nurse came in to tell us that the doctor would stop by in the morning with the imaging results. I got on the phone and called Judy to let her know that she needed to be there in the morning, then I sat beside my mother's bed and spent some quiet time just stroking her forehead while she dozed. When visiting hours were over, I kissed her goodnight and whispered that I'd be back early the next morning. I was reluctant to leave. Once back at her townhouse, I again set to work cleaning up the place until well after midnight.

By 7 A.M. I was in the busy hospital cafeteria picking up some fresh fruit that I thought might appeal to Mary Belle and perhaps brighten her spirits a bit. The "sitter," a different one this time, revealed that my mother had been "awake and combative" most of the night. It was disheartening news to receive. I'd hoped that that type of behavior had been left behind her.

Mom recognized me immediately. Her eyes lit up when she saw the fruit in my hands, yet she also began begging and pitifully pleading with me to get her out of there. Her words and especially the tone of her pleading pulled at my heart. It was emotionally difficult seeing her so stressed over her obvious sense of helplessness. She wanted out, yet no one was helping her to gain that one simple desire. It was hard on me knowing that she was expecting me to be her deliverer, when my hands were tied.

The doctor showed up around 10:30 A.M. and informed me that the MRI clearly showed cerebral atrophy consistent with her age and also some old lacunar infarcts (strokes), but no recent new ones. When I inquired about her recurring incidents of combative aggressiveness, he shrugged in puzzlement and regretfully admitted that he could not give me a definitive physiological reason for her current signs of dementia. His best guess was that it was most likely associated with the stress of having the cardiac catheterization done, coupled with her age, but, whatever the reason for it was, they were seriously considering moving her to the psychiatric unit the following day.

The doctor indirectly hinted at the necessity of the family giving serious consideration to doing a permanent nursing home placement for Mary Belle if the behavior continued to persist. At hearing this not-so-veiled suggestion, I realized that the situation was definitely not getting any brighter for my mother, yet I was standing in front of this doctor, thinking to myself, *Now just wait one minute. This lady was just fine before she got here, wasn't she? I'd just spoken to her on the phone the day before she was admitted and she had talked of her plans to drive down to Springfield to visit her sister. She'd never in her life been violent or aggressive. What did you do to my mother? How could this be happening?* I felt that I'd left Colorado and driven right across the border into the Twilight Zone.

My sister arrived while Mom was finishing her lunch and, after I filled her in on what the doctor had said, I was incredulous that she didn't have much of an opinion about what we'd been told and seemed to be perfectly okay with letting our mother go to the Psychiatric Unit. Mary Belle definitely did not want to go there. Since there was a difference of opinion on mother's next course of action, I left Judy with Mom for the duration of the evening visiting hours and returned to the townhouse to call Tony for his opinion.

Tony works as a computer programmer for a pharmaceutical research company in North Carolina and is highly familiarized with a wide range of drugs—drugs I'd never heard of. When I told him the drug names our mother was receiving, I was surprised to learn that the Trazodone and Haldol were both antipsychotics. I related to him that, as far as I was able to discern, our mother hadn't gotten more than two or three solid hours' sleep in any one twenty-four-hour period since I arrived, and that I thought that, perhaps, that element alone could certainly be a contributing factor to her uncharacteristic behavior. To make a long conversation short, we didn't take long to jointly decide on what to do next. He shared my opposition to placing mother in the Psychiatric Unit. I would get Mom discharged from the hospital tomorrow morning and bring her back to the townhouse for a couple of weeks while I could be right there with her to personally observe her behavior and reassess the entire disconcerting situation we'd all found ourselves in. We were family. We needed to work this out as a family unit. And, as a family, we'd journeyed to a critical crossroad that called for us to come to a mutually agreed-upon decision regarding the wisest manner in which to provide our mother with the best possible care and living arrangements to suit her special needs—needs that were, day by day, becoming more and more evident.

Before I informed the physician of our decision the following morning, I was half-expecting to be met with a challenge and had had all my mental ducks in a row in preparation for providing him with all of our reasons; yet my anticipation of a negative reaction from him was unfounded, for the doctor completely took me by surprise when he was quick to agree that our decision was a good idea, because "she very well might show some significant improvement in her own familiar home environment." On the other hand, he also seemed happy to be relieved of this troublesome patient and immediately made the necessary arrangements for a visiting nurse to stop by the house on a daily basis to monitor her blood pressure.

Much to Mary Belle's delight, we were out the hospital door before lunch, and, as soon as we were in the car, she animatedly asked if we could stop at Burger King. No problem. We went through the drive-through and then on home to reunite her with her beloved dog. She ate heartily and promptly fell into a deep sleep in her recliner until 9 P.M., when she awoke and wanted to take a shower. Afterward, I fixed us both some dinner, making a mental note to get to the grocery store in the morning.

This was now the 19th of October and the weatherperson on the television newscast was making more than a little noise about a possible storm building on the West Coast. Please, I silently begged, let the Snowmaker hold off a bit longer until I can get back home. A fall storm usually meant a possible (and probable) blizzard for our high Colorado location.

After dinner, we had a lengthy conversation and Mom repeatedly thanked me for getting her "out of there." She was visibly relieved to be back home, along with being physically exhausted from her ordeal. I tucked her in bed, Molly snuggled down at her feet, and she didn't wake again until 9 A.M. the next morning.

I guiltily felt lazy lying in bed at 7 A.M., and was still in my nightwear when I was startled by the front door being opened. To my great relief it was my sister's husband with a bag of fresh bagels in hand. I brewed us a fresh pot of coffee and we got a chance to visit together while Mom slept. Apparently, he'd been in the habit of stopping by with bagels for his "bagel buddy" every morning for quite some time. In talking with him though, I found out all sorts of disturbing things.

It seemed that Mary Belle hadn't been checked on as frequently as my brother and I had thought. Also, my brother-in-law informed me that Mary Belle had been doing things like getting lost while driving around the familiar territory of Shawnee Mission and had also driven through stop signs without even giving a thought to slowing down. I'd been concerned about Mom's driving as far back as last spring and had, more than once, tried suggesting to her that perhaps it was time to hang up her car keys, but both Mom and Judy had, at that time, insisted that she was doing "just fine" and my sister had promised me she'd keep a close eye out.

I also found out more things that Tony and I didn't know about. I was now informed that, one day, Mom had forgotten about some brownies she'd been baking and they burned in the oven. They'd actually caught on fire. She'd reached in to remove the pan with her bare hands.

Another newly revealed incident was when Mary Belle had taken the wrong medication by ingesting sleeping pills, when she thought she was taking her pain meds. I was absolutely incredulous that neither Tony nor I had been advised about these events that clearly placed my mother (and sometimes, others) in harmful situations.

Earlier in the year, Judy and I had discussed the possibility of her seventeen-year-old son moving in with Grandma, so she wouldn't be alone and he could be right there to help her with routine chores like getting in groceries and doing some light house upkeep. At the time, Mary Belle thought the plan was such a sure thing that she'd cleaned out the guest room closet and dresser drawers for him. But when six months had passed and he still hadn't made the move, Mom had been hurt over the entire situation.

Finally Mary Belle awoke and visited a bit with her son-in-law before he had to leave for an appointment. Mom and I spent the day knocking around the house—just being together. In the early afternoon, I called Judy to ask her to please come by and stay with Mother so I could get out to get the place stocked up on groceries.

Two days later, she found the time in her schedule to accommodate my request.

Being back in her home and having me there for company, Mary Belle was beginning to show great improvement. It's amazing what a little sound sleep and some nourishing down-home cooking can do. Also, I quit giving her the Haldol and Trazodone and just kept up with her blood pressure meds. I did make the addition of a good multiple vitamin with minerals and some extra B's to her daily regiment. Over the last year and a half, my mother had gone from a size 22 down to a 10. That's a lot of weight for someone her age to lose in that amount of time. When I questioned her about it, she denied having been on any kind of formal diet. My guess was that she'd, for whatever reason, simply lost interest in cooking for herself, as her appetite was certainly robust when I fixed her meals.

This was now her fourth day home from the hospital, and she'd shown no sign of aggressive behavior. Much to the contrary, she wanted to be active, get out and about, and visit her friends. When she excitedly mentioned this to the visiting nurse, we were duly informed in no uncertain terms that "if she left the house for any reason, the medical assistance would be discontinued." I thought this was absolutely ridiculous, because getting Mary Belle out was so good for her mental health. I was so sure of this that we conspired together and secretly sneaked out anyway. It was clearly evident that it did her a world of good.

I'd had several conversations with my sister about Mom's current living situation. After staying with Mary Belle and closely observing her behavior on a twenty-four-hour basis, I was completely convinced that she required some basic daily living assistance, due to the simple facts that she wouldn't ever think about eating unless I brought up the subject and also never remembered to take her medication. When I'd remind her, it was all too obvious that she wasn't quite sure which ones to take.

Judy, in seeing Mom's outward improvement since leaving the hospital, kept insisting that "Mary Belle would be just fine left alone in the townhouse." I couldn't believe that my sister couldn't seem to see the reality of our mother's desperately needful situation.

Observing Judy's continued perception and hearing her repeated pat response, I began to consider the strong possibility that she was playing mind games with herself and, perhaps subconsciously, didn't want to see it and had, therefore, conveniently placed herself in the comfortable and seemingly safe position of being in denial. I didn't know. All I had to go on was what I'd been observing. I knew that people had all sorts of different reactions to events in their lives and also various ways of dealing with them. I just didn't know where she was at because her perception of events appeared to be so much different from Tony's and mine. She just didn't want to discuss the possibility that something was wrong in our mother's life, and that the time had come when alternate courses needed to be set for her.

I had, by this time, been away from Colorado for a week and a half and knew I needed to help Mom deal with her situation before I returned home. It was clear to me that the status of her current living conditions (lifestyle) was not satisfactory for her any longer. She was in no physical or mental condition to be left to her own devices and, after all I'd recently learned and observed, I couldn't count on her being alright without closer monitoring. In desperation and total frustration, I called Tony and asked him to fly out to Kansas City and help me decide on some alternate arrangements for our mother. He readily agreed and said he'd be there on Friday.

This was my mother's life, and I in no way wanted to make her decisions for her. Consequently, she and I spent a great deal of time exploring and discussing her options for alternative living arrangements. It was a great relief to me when she freely admitted to the fact that she recognized and understood the reality of her situation, that she needed help with daily living. She confided to me that she'd frequently been scared living alone in the townhouse and also needed help keeping her bills straight and meals fixed. She confessed that she'd had a "few" small fires in the oven and on the stovetop. She openly expressed an awareness (and disappointment) that, more and more, her memory seemed to be failing. She also suspected that these disconcerting events were not all attributed to her previous strokes, because she'd noticed that her former ability to verbalize thoughts was becoming more and more difficult to manage.

It was clear that my mother was adamant about the *fact* that she would *not* go to a nursing home because, among the obvious reasons, she couldn't take her dog with her and I wholeheartedly agreed. I would feel the same way. The alternate choices were few. Tony was currently residing in an apartment in North Carolina and was engaged to be married soon. Judy and her husband lived in Kansas City (where Mom preferred to stay, of course), but my sister also had four children in a three-bedroom house. I, on the other hand, lived in Colorado with my friend, Mary, in a two-bedroom cabin and could give my bedroom completely over to Mary Belle; yet, that option would also remove her from her friends and grandchildren. Every available option Mom and I examined appeared to have drawbacks. There was no singular, perfect solution to our dilemma. We felt like we were spinning our wheels trying to find that one, elusive resolution.

Just down the street from mother's church, a new "assisted living" facility was sketched out on the drawing board. Though the builders hadn't even broken ground for it yet, Mary Belle liked the idea and seemed to think that she could manage living alone there. Although I did somewhat placate her by calling the organization for the particulars on the various types of apartments being offered, and actually went as far as placing her name on the waiting list, in my heart I didn't foresee this as being a true option for her. It wasn't a viable option because of the prohibitive annual cost and the fact that it didn't provide the greater level of assistance my mother now required. In the end, things were looking as though the best option for her was to come back to Colorado to live with me and, after closely looking at every conceivable alternative and discussing all facets of them, surprisingly enough, she was eagerly agreeing with the Colorado scenario. She even went as far as going into her room and digging out her cowboy hat to prove that she was indeed ready to "head for the hills."

Our discussions that night were thorough ones. They also included the realities of such important issues as an updated will, power of attorney documents, and the Do Not Resuscitate orders that she'd previously written. Mom and I got on the phone with Tony that evening and discussed all that she and I had explored together in the comfort of her living room. He quickly agreed that Colorado was her best choice of all the options. In that same conversation with him, Mary Belle requested that Tony and I share power of attorney for her and her estate, and assist her in making the plans to sell her townhouse.

Finally, finally, it felt as though something solid was beginning to take shape and I was greatly relieved because, up to this point, I had been unable to get Judy to participate in helping us come to any kind of decision in regard to our mother's pressing situation, and some decisions definitely needed to be made without any further delays. More than anything, I wanted whole family participation in this important process. Instead, Judy continued to hold her ground, wanting me to return to Colorado and leave everything as I'd found it—in a status quo state. Tony and I knew that her alternative was not one of the options.

My mother was asking for help from her children. There was no way I was going to turn a deaf ear to that soulful call.

After our conference call with Tony, Mom gently set her cowboy hat on the dining room table (so she wouldn't forget

to wear it in the morning) and, with a sweet smile of gratitude, went off to bed. She looked so tired, yet seemed excited
about the thought of moving to the mountains. Her relief at
finally reaching a decision was evident.

With her in bed, I now had some time to myself and, in
that privacy, I called my friend Mary to let her know that the
previous stagnant situation was finally experiencing some
progression. She was glad to hear that. We'd previously discussed the entire situation and, being a deeply compassionate person, she didn't hesitate a second over exuberantly
supporting the idea of bringing my mother into our cabin to
live. Though I'd been reticent to point out how small our
place was, and that her cherished solitude would probably
no longer be what it was, and the peace and quiet that was
needed for her research and writing would most likely be
seriously compromised, I voiced those negative elements
anyway. All she did was reiterate her solid support and
emphasize the fact that she didn't see how we could do anything else because "it was the spiritual thing to do." With
her, any decision needing to be made always came down to
asking oneself "what is the most *spiritual* thing to do?" In
other words, what choice represents the most ethical,
humanitarian, or moral one to make?

Her answer echoed my own feelings, and it was so incredibly comforting for me to know that my mother would be a
truly welcomed addition to our serene and tranquil mountain
home. Although Mary understood that we'd also be bringing
another dog into the family unit, it presented no problem for
her—no problem at all because she well knew and fully understood the great emotional impact that four-legged compan-
ions could have on people. I also told her that I was aware that
the newscasters were predicting heavy snowfall for the coming week in Colorado and that I'd have to really hustle to
finalize everything that needed to be done if I wanted to beat
the forecast storm. She responded with, "Please don't rush on
my account. I'll be just fine." Although I heard her words, I

also felt my own inner promptings, which strongly urged me to put a "rush order" on that hustle.

The following morning I put in a call to my friend Stephanie who worked for a prestigious local law firm as a legal assistant. I explained my situation to her. She admitted that she didn't have all the answers to my immediate questions, but would be glad to find out and get right back to me.

My next call was to an old family friend who was a real estate agent. I learned that she'd recently retired, so I was referred to a friend of hers. The wheels were in motion by the time Judy stopped by that afternoon. In fact, those wheels were spinning so fast that the Realtor actually walked in the door while I was trying to explain Mom's recent decisions to my sister. It was a tense moment, to say the least, and I had to ask Judy to come back later, as I had paperwork to sign for getting Mom's place listed.

Judy returned an hour later and was not pleased with the way things were going. She made the comment that I was "just coming in and taking over," all the while insisting that Mom was "just fine and didn't need any interference from me in her life."

Well, my sister and the rest of the family were obviously not going to agree on that point, so I asked Mary Belle to sit down with us and talk to Judy herself. Again, for Judy's sake, I attempted to come up with some alternate options to ease my sister's concern over taking our mother out of Kansas City. When I suggested the very viable option of taking the proceeds from the townhouse sale and either purchasing Judy a larger home with an attached mother-in-law quarters or simply adding on an apartment with a bedroom, den, and small kitchen/bath to her existing home for Mary Belle, my sister gave us a nonplussed look of exasperation and said that she'd have to talk it over with her husband. I was trying to give her an opportunity to take advantage of a couple of possible ways to keep her mother near her. But my suggestion never went any further than being just a suggestion that didn't receive any serious consideration.

At that same time, I'd also asked Judy for any ideas on what she thought might best benefit our mother and nothing was forthcoming. Everything I would suggest was somehow not good, but she herself offered absolutely nothing as a compromise or alternative. By declining to make suggestions or contribute her constructive suggestions regarding the decisions that Mary Belle, Tony, and I had to make, she literally forced us to make them without her input. Granted, every possible solution required compromises, yet she seemed unwilling to place herself in a position of accepting any compromise the rest of us saw as being necessary.

Once several of the major decisions were solidified, Mom got out her suitcases and started packing while wearing her cowboy hat. If the situation hadn't been so tangled in the psychological issues of family conflict, it would've been funny to see Mom help pack up her things while wearing that hat. This would only be her third move and thinning out her massive accumulation of a lifetime of possessions was a daunting undertaking. The job was left to her and me to accomplish together.

Finally it was time to call about renting a moving van, and I made arrangements to pick one up the following Sunday. Tony would be in town then and, thankfully, would be available to help me load it, as I was beginning to see I couldn't count on anyone else to offer their help in getting this job done. Grandma had been home from the hospital for more than a week now and no one had come by to visit her. I was incredulous over that, but, fortunately, far too busy to dwell on it.

My mother's closets were full of clothing articles that no longer fit her and we had to sort through every one. The massive china cabinet was packed with dishes, linens, games, and a wide variety of crystal and silver specialty pieces. With stuff everywhere, a decision had to be made about every little item in the place. It was an enormous and exhausting undertaking to sort it all out, because I was continually asking Mary Belle, "What do you want to do with this? If you don't want that knickknack, who do you want to give it to?"

Mom ended up choosing to take only those items that held emotional attachments for her and decided to leave all the rest, including her massive eight-foot-long china hutch, the entire living room set, the Ethan Allen dining set, washer and dryer, one bedroom set, kitchen contents, and the good china, to Judy. There was still an incredible amount designated for the moving van; a favorite antique lyre-table with marble top, a tall free-standing rotating bookcase, and boxes upon boxes of precious knickknacks along with seventy-nine years' worth of cherished memorabilia. So, for the rest of the week I was kept busy packing, packing, and packing some more. Day and night I made piles for different designations, so, by the time Tony arrived in town, the house was a mountain of boxes with narrow walking paths cleared between them all.

The night before Tony arrived, Judy finally came over around 10 P.M. She and I spent the entire night talking and crying in our efforts to smooth out our differences and make up. As the sun was rising she came over and hugged me, telling me that she was sorry for remaining distant through the whole thing.

While I'd been busy packing up my mother's house in Kansas City, a massive snow system had been equally busy dumping four feet of snow with five- and six-foot-high drifts against the walls of the little Colorado cabin. I didn't beat the predicted storm as I'd hoped. When I called Mary, she said she'd been shoveling round the clock just trying to keep a small area clear so the dogs could go outside and she could keep the weight off the 35-by-15-foot deck to keep it from collapsing.

As mentioned previously, our driveway leading down to the cabin is one-quarter mile long and runs downhill from the road. We have an old Jeep and a plow blade but Mary doesn't drive a stick shift and also doesn't have the physical strength it takes to maneuver the gearshift and the blade operation. Our friends Marcia and Jim had attempted to dig her out with their plow, but couldn't manage to get into the drive more than twenty yards from the road. The snow had fallen too fast and, with the whipping winds, drifted too high in places for them to break through the wet, heavy barriers.

Mary was snowed in and completely isolated from the rest of the world. She had plenty of food, gasoline and oil for the generator, and firewood for heat, but would be in trouble if she needed any kind of medical assistance. She informed me that, fortunately, the phone was still operable and friends and her daughters had been calling several times a day to check on her. But this weather situation back home greatly intensified the urgency and anxiety I was feeling to return to Colorado. I had two major responsibilities, and they were 700 miles apart from each other.

When I again spoke with Mary on the phone she'd exclaimed that, in the twenty years she'd been living in Colorado, she'd never seen such fierce, howling winds with a blizzard. It seemed that they were haphazardly blustering and whipping in from all directions. In her attempt to ease my stress level, she kept insisting that she was perfectly okay and that I shouldn't worry about her. Though it may have been my imagination, I wasn't sure that was what I was hearing in her voice. Later, I discovered that what I'd picked up on was concern over my drive back through the snow in the moving van with the car in tow.

The following day was Saturday, and my friend Stephanie from the law office came over with all the pertinent legal documents we needed. She, Tony, Mary Belle, and I sat down and got them signed and notarized in an hour's time. Stephanie was a godsend, and I owe her a debt of gratitude for handling the legal powers of attorney and living will papers.

Tony and I picked up the moving van with the attached tow dolly for my car on Sunday morning. Afterwards we went to a furniture store to pick up the two new recliners Mary Belle had bought for herself during one of our secret outings together: one for the cabin's living room and one for her new bedroom. Previously, mother had been using an old worn one that'd been purchased in the early 70s and was not worth hauling to the dump. I wanted her to have comfortable personal furniture items in her new Colorado home, especially something for her to use in the privacy of her bedroom, where she could watch television, read, or just sit back and doze.

Back at the townhouse, Tony and I started loading up the truck. Eventually, after we were nearly finished, Judy's husband and a couple of his teenaged boys showed up to help. The snowstorm that had dumped on Colorado had blown its way into Kansas, and the rain it pushed in front of it was hard and steady. We worked fast and furious trying not to get Mother's possessions drenched while making our way with them from the house to the van. Just as we closed the van door, the rain turned into driving sheets.

Eventually, on Grandma's last night in town, Judy's kids made their way over to visit her. Tony ran out for burgers and the "family" sat around for the rest of the evening. Mother had given most of her larger furniture pieces to Judy, so those were about the only items left scattered here and there around the house.

Tony finally had to leave for the airport to fly back to North Carolina and Judy took her kids home around ten o'clock.

Tired, Mom and I went straight to bed as soon as everyone left.

At the crack of dawn, she was up and eager to begin her big Colorado adventure, and we were out of the house by 5 A.M.

In the cab of the van Mom was excited. With her cowboy hat on and her dog lying across her lap, she was anxious to be heading for those forested hills of the high country. It was still pouring rain and the wipers on the truck were being spastic. Neither she nor I cared; we both wanted out of Kansas City.

With the fully loaded van pulling my old Corolla behind it, we did well to get up to 60 m.p.h. once in a while, so it was already a long trip even before we hit the wall of snow that still held Colorado in its crippling grip. In some places we were literally driving through tunnels of snow made by the state plows and we couldn't see beyond either side of the snowy walls.

I kept an eye on Mary Belle to gauge how she was handling the long drive. She slept for several hours and was doing fairly well, so I decided to try and push it all the way home, rather than stopping at a motel.

We crossed the Kansas border.

We reached Limon, Colorado.

Then Colorado Springs.

Woodland Park. And darkness fell.

I stopped in Divide to phone Mary to let her know of the good progress we'd made. The relief in her voice to hear that we were only fifteen minutes from home was unmistakable. She informed me that two of our friends had hiked in the day before and had managed to open up the drive with our Jeep. They'd been able to plow it just enough for me to make it through with the moving van. The timing couldn't have been closer.

It was nightfall when I finally pulled onto the drive and it was all downhill through the narrowly opened ribbon of cleared snow. The pathway twisted down and around through the dark woods until we reached the point where the cabin's exterior floodlights helped to light the way. We slipped and slid a bit, but, being so elated by finally arriving safely at our destination, we felt as if Ezekiel's team itself was pulling us through, as we slowly rolled to a stop at the back garden gate.

Home. We were *home.*

Though Mom was clearly excited, she was also dead tired. We got her right up to bed without any argument. Mary had my bedroom all prepared for its new occupant and Mom quickly fell fast asleep between clean crisp sheets. The heat from the living room woodstove rose up the stairwell and filled the loft-like room with air warm as toast.

My friend and I then had time to sit down in the living room to talk. The reality of the situation was just starting to sink in for me. At forty-three years of age, I was once again "living with my mother."

What had I done? The entire experience in Kansas City had definitely seemed like it'd been some kind of scenario right out of an old *Twilight Zone* episode—no reality there (or perhaps too much), but now, sitting face to face with Mary in our small living room, with the delicate fragrance of her cedar incense filling the air and the fire in the stove crackling, made my recent actions a growing realization. What had I done? This was her home, too. The reality of it was evolving into something that teetered between horror and necessity. I did what I had to do.

For the most part over the years, I'd been the one sibling to mow mother's yard, repair her plumbing, fix her roof, take her on vacations after my father passed away. Wasn't it someone else's turn? And what of my friend Mary, who had only briefly met my mother once before, when we'd stayed at her house during a cross-country book-signing tour? How was she going to eventually come to feel about having "my family" in our cabin on a permanent basis?

The full ramifications were hitting me hard in respect to how they might affect my friend—my friend who'd been admirably recuperating from her own life's personal griefs, and now I'd taken away her peace and solitude by bringing my mother into our home. My head was spinning with a jumble of thoughts. Oh God, give us strength. What had I done?

The following day, our same friends returned to help us out. They arrived early in the morning to assist in unloading the van. Actually, they had the truck 95 percent empty and cartons distributed to their respective areas of the cabin before I realized it.

During those days when Mary had been snowed in by herself, she'd been busier than a squirrel gathering nuts in late autumn, making the appropriate cabin arrangements to accommodate my mother's arrival. She'd completely emptied my closet and cleared out my dresser and bookshelves to make places for Mary Belle to put her own possessions. She'd stored some of her own things away to make room for my clothing in her closet and dresser drawers. I literally had no bedroom now, and Mary had thoughtfully distributed many of my personal things about the cabin, so that I wouldn't feel completely displaced. In the living room, she'd rearranged the furniture to make room for the recliner I'd told her we were bringing in for Mary Belle. To this day I don't know how she maneuvered the heavy furniture by herself and managed to clear areas all over the house, so Mom would have prominent places to set out her own personal belongings. Mary had made a huge pile of her own possessions, designated for Goodwill, down in the basement, just to make room for my Mom's incoming stuff. Other than being happy to see her personal "things" come out of the packing boxes, my mother didn't seem to notice or realize all the work Mary had gone to so that she could feel welcome and truly "at home." Mary, of course, never said a word about it.

The truck was due back the following day and I got it halfway up the drive before I began having difficulty. Being empty and needing to go uphill in the packed snow, it began backsliding toward a large aspen. I left it in the middle of the drive and walked back to call a tow truck. When the driver arrived, he took one critical look at the situation, got in the moving van and, without a pause, drove it right up the drive. Guess I was just too worn out by then to realize that I could've done the same thing myself.

Now that the move was made, there were a million and one details to attend to. One of the first orders of business was filling out dozens of change-of-address notices for Mary Belle. Because of the security issue we're presented with by Mary being an internationally known author, we'd always had an unlisted telephone number. Now, we were faced with making it more public for my mother's benefit. All of her friends and relatives were sent the address and phone number. I felt as though our former privacy had been terribly invaded by this "social expectation" by others, but also knew that I could do nothing else.

The following weeks were relegated to getting the last of the boxes unpacked. And, since my mother had always been used to having her own desk, I emptied out my small, oak rolltop, and Mary and I carried it up into Mom's bedroom.

Next came the search for new doctors for Mom. Mary obtained a recommendation for a cardiologist in Colorado Springs from one of her doctor friends, and we also used the general practitioner here in Cripple Creek. Mom and I were able to bring her medical records with us from Kansas City, which proved to be a great help. I made her an appointment.

The cardiologist checked her over and, after suggesting that I concentrate on just "keeping her comfortable," said to come back for a checkup every six months. The doctor in Cripple Creek wanted to get her started on Gingko biloba, a variety of extra vitamins, and also B-12 shots in an effort to help improve her memory.

Mary Belle was emotionally invigorated by the extra attention she was receiving along with three square meals a day and eight hours of solid sleep each night. She was a new woman. So, with her renewed interest in life, she and I started discussing adding alternative health options to supplement her traditional treatments. She decided she'd like to try acupuncture. I called a doctor friend of ours, and she referred us to a wonderful woman in Colorado Springs. We started with weekly appointments, and some of mother's physical complaints and symptoms eased.

The next thing I did was purchase her a membership in the Cripple Creek Beach and Yacht Club (a humorous name since this is a high mountain mining town with no body of water in sight) at the Holiday Inn Express motel, so she could go into their pool several times a week. She'd always greatly enjoyed being in a pool and I thought that this activity, in conjunction with using the hot tub Jacuzzi for her arthritis, would be a highly enjoyable and physically therapeutic activity for her to indulge herself in.

Mary and I had taken a day to go down to Colorado Springs and purchase nearly $200 worth of puzzles, games, and activity projects from Hobby Lobby for Mary Belle to keep occupied with. We also bought her a maple table for her to work her projects on. Suddenly I found that I was devoting four and five days each week just to handling Mary Belle's business.

As the weeks passed, it was becoming clear that living on a generator presented a safety problem for my mother. She kept forgetting all the various ways we needed to alter the normal ways of doing daily (and nightly) things. She'd go downstairs during the night and walk about in the dark cabin. If I wasn't such a deep sleeper, I'd have heard her, but even being on the couch, I'd only wake up after Mary had come downstairs at 3 A.M., and there was a commotion with Mary Belle not wanting Mary to lead her back up to bed. Although Mary and I had never planned on getting connected to the power grid, we now had no choice in the matter if we wanted to keep Mary Belle safe. The luxury of the power grid being our option was taken from us. One of the many reasons we didn't want power run down the road was that it'd increase the value of the adjacent land we'd hoped to someday purchase. Now we had no choice in the matter. We contacted the power company.

Once the power line was installed underground to the cabin the following May, we gifted my mother with a small aquarium for her room and bought the Dish Network cable service to give her "viewing options," and had a separate line run to her television so she could watch whatever she wanted in the privacy of her own room.

The next unanticipated problem to raise its head was the apparent stress and strain that the stairs were causing Mary Belle. They were extremely tiring for her, and she'd begun to ascend them on all fours and make her descent by slowly lowering herself while sitting down on one step at a time. She had a serious heart condition, but also had previously undergone an operation to have both knees replaced. This situation constantly concerned Mary and me, and, after spending a great deal of time trying to discover a solution, I came up with a workable resolution that would make it completely unnecessary for her to ever again have a need to use the stairs. I thought of the same idea I'd formerly posed to Judy for her own house—that of using a bit of mother's money to add on a separate, private ground floor bedroom and bath for her convenience.

Mary wasn't sold on the idea of using my mother's money to do that, but, since we'd never planned on adding on another bed and bath in the future for ourselves, and she could see the stress those stairs were having on Mary Belle, she was okay with the idea because it wouldn't be a self-serving use of someone else's money.

I first posed the option to my mother and she liked the idea a lot. She liked the idea of having her own living "quarters" rather than just one bedroom to herself. I then wanted to have the rest of the family's okay for the plan because I didn't want to do something that major without their concurring opinion. One had no objection. One did. And the family suddenly found itself with a major issue to argue over.

Mary, who had eventually grown disgusted with the ongoing conflict within my family, finally put her foot down and ended the heated debate by flatly refusing to add onto the cabin. "Enough is enough," she'd said. "Let it go."

And we did. I have to honestly admit, though I hadn't realized what my family had been doing—that my own family was actually arguing over what to do with a cabin that Mary was part-owner of—I was relieved that the incredible stress of the problem was finally lifted from all concerned.

So now that Mary Belle had no choice but to contend with the problem of the stairs, Mary and I attempted to reduce the physical stress of the situation by limiting Mother's use of them. We'd run up and down to get Mother various things she wanted from her bedroom during the day.

Finally, after she began roaming downstairs and out into the woods during the middle of the night, we had to install a makeshift Dutch door type of barrier gate at the top of the stairs to keep her from sneaking down when we were asleep. When she found a way around that by crawling underneath the door, I had to add spaced panels to the bottom of it. This greatly angered Mary Belle. While watching me install the additional panels she sarcastically said, "Now look what you've gone and done. That's really, really *ugly*. You made your place look awful!"

I replied that I agreed, but also reminded her that I wouldn't have had to do it if she'd only stay in her room at night and not sneak outside. That rationale didn't seem to sink in because she still wanted out when she wanted out—even if it was three in the morning—so, thereafter, she'd stand at the top of the stairs kicking at the boards and rattling the gate until she woke the entire household, and we either rationally talked her down from her agitation or had to physically guide her back into her room.

Shortly after the installation of the makeshift safety gate, Mary Belle began having night "incidents" which necessitated my immediate response to her and the locked gate that hampered my response time became a new problem. Consequently, another adjustment to our lives became evident—I could no longer be asleep downstairs and also get up to my mother as quickly as I sometimes needed to with a locked gate between us. In order to resolve this dilemma I had no choice but to ask her if I could sleep in her bedroom recliner during the night. That request didn't go over well at all. "Absolutely not," she'd said, "this is *my* room!" Okay then, the only alternative was to sleep in the recliner in Mary's room, which was just across the hall.

At the outset of Mary Belle's arrival, Mary had been sympathetic and deeply concerned that I no longer had any private space in the house to call my own, that I no longer had a room of my own in my own home. Now that circumstances proved that a locked gate between Mary Belle (upstairs) and me (downstairs) during the night hampered my ability to get to her quickly enough, my friend had no problem at all with me camping out in the recliner in her room at night.

Our lives were continually changing.

Also, it wasn't long before we realized that the activity projects we'd bought Mom, like the puzzles, games, and needlework pieces, were useless. One evening when the three of us sat down at the kitchen table to play Monopoly (one of the games we'd bought for her because she'd always enjoyed playing it), she began throwing the houses and hotels across the board instead of the dice. Card games, too, even the simplest types, such as Go Fish, were far too complicated to play at her declining level of mental ability. The new puzzles were fun for her up to a point—only until all the straight-edged border pieces were found and fit together to make the frame, but after that, it was far too difficult for her to manage, and, frustrated, she quickly lost interest in them (other than to check to see how Mary and I were progressing on our work of finishing them up for her). So we found that she could only work puzzles with fifty pieces or less, and Mary Belle gave all her newly acquired needlework projects to Mary and me. In addition, reading had become too complex an activity to hold her interest, as we'd catch her "pretending" to read magazine articles and books. To the casual observer it would appear that she was indeed deeply engrossed in her literary material, yet, upon closer inspection, that same observer would soon notice that Mary Belle was either reading from back to front, or that she was dozing, or that the book was upside down.

I've noticed that several times mother will "pretend" to be doing something that she is no longer capable of. She's gotten really expert at faking out those who call her on the telephone by simply letting them carry the bulk of the conversation while she makes noncommittal and very vague, nonspecific statements such as, "how nice" or "oh really, isn't that great" when she can't remember the personal facts that the other individual expects her to. She's fooled several people, who will then turn around and say to me, "Mary Belle sounds perfectly fine to me." Hearing that kind of comment or opinion gives the caregiver the distinct sense that people on the outside think you're exaggerating her condition and don't quite believe you. This situation is commonly experienced by the at-home caregiver and can become quite frustrating. Oh yes, at that point my mother was so "fine" that she couldn't even write her own name without having me first write it down in order for her to copy it.

General behavior, too, became erratic and more uncharacteristic of my mother's normal personality. My mother had always been a highly intelligent person, formerly working for a major financial institution, where she'd personally prepared the tax returns of Bess Truman (wife of former President Truman), among other notable individuals. Now she couldn't even make heads or tails of her checking account statement, write a check, or even remember how to spell her name when signing greeting cards.

This new situation left all of her financial affairs to me, and, although I was glad to handle them for her, she soon began to exhibit a completely irrational and unfounded paranoia, and sometimes had it in her head that I was stealing her money—this last notion being a commonly recognized and noted symptom evidenced with most Alzheimer's patients. Still, it was heartbreaking for me to hear my own mother accusing me of ridiculous things when I (and Mary) had readjusted our entire lives around her and found ourselves devoting so much of our personal time giving attention to her increasing needs and various affairs. We never expected to receive recognition or appreciation for these ongoing readjustments we made, but neither did we expect to be the focus of her unfounded suspicions and be the subjects of her complaints to family and friends whenever she spoke to them on the telephone. What was just as incredible was that there were those who were immediately ready to believe her and accept her accusations as hard fact!

Other evidence of suspiciousness surfaced when she began standing directly in front of Mary or myself whenever we received a personal phone call—thinking that the call was actually for her and then continually motioning for us to hand over the receiver so she could speak. She was absolutely convinced that every time the phone rang it was for her. Whenever one of Mary's daughters or friends called or, more importantly, whenever one of her many publishing business contacts called, such as various department heads from Hampton Roads Publishing Company, or from her editor at Pocket Books, or from her foreign rights agent at Writer's House in New York, she had no privacy at all because my mother would be right there, standing not more than five feet away from her—intently listening to every single word being said. If any part of the conversation Mary was having involved the issue of money, my mother thought it was about *her* money and, later, demanded to know where *her* check was.

I never dreamed that, by bringing Mother into our home, so much of our personal space would be taken away. I don't mean physical space, but rather the "space of individual privacy." We soon had no privacy whatsoever in our home and were forced to resort to actions such as taking the phone down into the basement in order to talk to people without her listening to everything said and then misconstruing it. This simple effort to gain some precious privacy only intensified her delusional conviction that we were "conspiring together and keeping her calls from her."

Whenever one of those previously mentioned necessities arose, when it was imperative for both Mary and me to be away from the house at the same time for some type of joint errand or mutual appointment, we'd return to immediately notice that both of our desks had been rifled through and, frequently, important documents such as bills were missing from Mary's rolltop—Mother had taken them and hidden them from us thinking that they were hers and was planning to use them as "proof" that we were spending her money. Mary tends to be an extremely efficient and orderly individual. Everything has a place. She can spot a pencil on her desk that's been moved out of place. And once, quite to my friend's complete and utter dismay, we'd returned home to find that my mother had ripped seven pages of Mary's research notes related to one of her current book projects out of a notepad and had hidden those too. My mother had sequestered them so well that we tore the house apart and never found them. When questioned, Mary Belle completely denied touching a thing while we were gone. Denial to avoid culpability is a common Alzheimer's trait. Luckily, though, Mary was able to recall most of what she'd written down and, by the following morning, had successfully reconstructed all of the notes by memory. Now Mary had to expend the extra time and effort of hiding all of her works-in-progress to protect them from vanishing, not to mention all our personal papers and important, irreplaceable documents related to the property and her business.

Another strange behavioral trait we encountered was a situation involving my mother's eating habits. Mary Belle would not eat unless the meal was prepared by Mary or myself and placed directly in front of her. Though mother was strongly reassured time and again that the kitchen was as much hers as ours, and that she should always feel free to take whatever she wanted to eat from the cupboards or fridge whenever she felt like eating a meal or just snacking on this or that, she would not voluntarily make the effort to get herself as little as a cup of coffee or remove a sweet roll from its packaging, but then she'd get on the phone with people and we'd overhear her telling family members and her personal friends that she *"wasn't being fed."* Incidents like that just made me want to scream and pull out my hair because, in actuality, whenever Mary and I went down into Woodland Park to do the grocery shopping, we'd purposely purchased all manner of extra food items for Mother—items that we wouldn't have normally purchased—items that were those quick and easy-to-fix foodstuffs just to accommodate my mother's ease of serving herself.

Also, during this same time frame she began to believe that both of us were continually lying to her, and we discovered that this happened only because she couldn't remember events or what was said three minutes beforehand.

Whenever Mary and I would be gone from the house for just a short time, we had to resort to turning off the telephone bell ringer and hiding the portable receiver because, if we didn't, Mary Belle would busy herself by calling long-distance wrong numbers, she'd even once called 911 to "talk to the nicest lady there." Also, she would intercept Mary's business calls, and heaven only knows what she said to whom.

Other problems arose whenever we'd both be away from the cabin at the same time. My mother began doing things like letting our dogs out the wrong door and they'd be loose in the woods instead of within the safety of their dog yard (this is serious because most of our dogs are very small Yorkies—a couple of them smaller than the average size for the breed—and there are coyotes, hawks, bears, and owls in our woods). One afternoon we returned home to the acrid smell of burnt toast permeating the cabin and discovered that the toaster dial had been turned all the way up and she'd told us that she'd tried to extract her piece of toast with a knife. Another time when we returned from being gone only twenty minutes, the flame was flaring on high on the propane kitchen range top.

These incidents (and many more like them) were telling. They made it crystal clear to us that leaving Mary Belle alone in the house was a highly dangerous thing to do. We could no longer leave the cabin together to go anywhere unless we had a "respite" person to sit for my mother during our absence. We couldn't even leave her alone long enough to make the ten-minute drive up to the post office to pick up our mail. For us, there was no more social life—no more going out in the evenings, no more going to baby showers or parties, or shopping—without taking Mary Belle along, no more coming home in the wee hours of the morning after a night out with friends. This new situation completely altered our lives as one of us always had to be home. Consequently, for us to get out together (mostly for a break) we now had to pay someone for this "respite" care service at least twice a week. This is not the same as paying a teenaged babysitter. It is definitely not the same at all. It's paying a professional and that professional's services are very costly.

Finally, Mary Belle's physician officially diagnosed my mother with Alzheimer's, and, after hearing about all the typical behavioral patterns that both Mary and I had observed Mary Belle exhibiting, he didn't hesitate to shake his head and say, "You two shouldn't have to put up with this constant aggravation. You both have your own lives to live. I strongly recommend placing your mother in a nursing home."

As soon as his attending nurse heard him make these strong statements, she took the cue to go next door to check the attached Hilltop Nursing Home for vacancies. While she was gone from the room, I told him, "no way." I told him that, early on, when I'd been having problems with my sister about bringing Mom out to Colorado, I'd checked into that option in Kansas City, and the cost was prohibitive ($25,000 to $35,000 and up per year for full-time, full care). "And, anyway," I added, "I want my mother to live at home with familiar family around her until the end." I reminded him that "although her behavior and thought process have greatly altered, she's still my mother, and I love her just as much now as I always have in spite of her continually altering personality and behavior." I informed him that my mother, in her more lucid days, had always been extremely adamant about her desire to live at home rather than at a nursing home.

As it happened, the Hilltop Nursing Home didn't accept patients with Alzheimer's who "roamed" and required full care in a "locked" facility.

The singular remaining loose end that I still had to attend to was how to get mother's 1986 Chevy Nova out to Colorado. I'd asked my sister if she or one of her sons could drive it out from Kansas and Mary's daughter's fiancé could fly him back (he pilots small planes). No, that wasn't acceptable to her because she doesn't trust the small planes. So then we offered to personally pay for a commercial airline ticket to fly him back. No, that wasn't acceptable either because, although her eldest son was eighteen and currently preparing to go off to college, her reasoning was that he'd never driven that far by himself before. So once again the responsibility fell on me to take care of it. I flew to Kansas City and drove the vehicle back, registered it with the State of Colorado and did the paperwork to get Mother the handicapped plates she'd previously had on it.

In every reference book I've researched on Alzheimer's (and I bought a slew of them), it appears that this disease, more than any other, presents convoluted, psychological familial elements, especially when one family member is the primary at-home caregiver. Mary and I have witnessed this firsthand and seen this to be valid. Although the caregiver does everything within her/his power to provide safe and healthful care to the afflicted loved one, there will always be one (or more) family member who is either in denial or in continual conflict over that care— usually because they have no idea of the severity of mental decline taking place, the psychological machinations that the patient exhibits, or the incredible amount of additional daily work and stress this can create for the devoted caregiver.

My mother has been with Mary and me for more than three years now and the rapid decline we've seen in her mental state has been nothing less than dramatic and astounding. Although we've managed to maintain her physical health through nourishing meals, medication, routine blood pressure monitoring, and exercise, her mental state has sunk into the ever-deepening dementia stages of Alzheimer's. My brother, my mother's sister, and Mary's daughters have been extremely supportive of what we did daily for my mother.

I want to express my deepest appreciation to my friend Mary for so readily welcoming my mother into our home, for graciously accepting the fact that the serenity of our cabin has been seriously compromised, and for continually putting up with the incredibly frustrating and frequently exasperating behavioral symptoms of an elder with late-stage Alzheimer's.

Between us, as twenty-four-hour caregivers, we've managed to show Mary Belle that she was loved, that in her mountain home, love never sleeps. Although in her deepening dementia she didn't always understand that, we sincerely believe that, on some level within the core of her being, she knew it was true. I love my mother. I always will.

II. The Classic Clinical Behavioral Symptoms of Alzheimer's Disease and their Management by the At-Home Caregiver

$\mathcal{L}oss$ of $Cognition$

The loss of cognition (rationale, logic, and memory) is most often the first noticeable symptom evidenced with Alzheimer's disease. This symptom includes such behavioral evidence as moments of sudden confusion, disassociative thought patterns, an inability to follow conversation, diminished attention span, increasing forgetfulness, a loss of concentration and mental focus, suddenly not recognizing familiar places or people, waning verbal communication skills (not being able to speak the right word associated with a thought, or the substitution of completely unrelated terms), and making disconnected statements, which are frequently illogical or appear nonsensical.

This singular initial, multifaceted symptom is a subtle one that has the tendency to creep up on the unaware individual, because we all experience those disconcerting times when we stride with purpose into a room and then, dumbfounded, stand there scratching our heads in wonderment as we suddenly realize that we forgot why we were headed there in the first place. We all have forgotten where the car keys were placed, have had events in our lives when we couldn't remember a frequently called phone number—maybe even our own—or have forgotten an important occasion such as a son's or daughter's wedding anniversary. These simple lapses of memory are common and, therefore, are why the initial Alzheimer's symptom of "loss of cognition" is so easily masked and goes undetected.

It's an extremely subtle symptom which, over time, increases in frequency and prevents the early recognition of it as being a valid warning bell that loudly peals out the signal that something more than "normal forgetfulness" is at work. Because of this natural human tendency to nonchalantly attribute "normalcy" to these occurrences, it's easy for family members to remain in denial over a parent's increasing loss of their various types of cognitive skills. It's easy to quickly comment, "Oh, dad's okay; it's just old age, just all a part of growing old." But it's not always so. That's been proven to not always be the case. I personally know several elderly people who, in their late 80s, are as mentally sharp as a tack and lead intellectually fulfilling and physically active lives. They study, jog, attend lectures, travel overseas for leisure, actively maintain all of their personal financial affairs including various investments, keep up the maintenance of several homes, etc. Growing old is not a death sentence for one's mind. *Aging, in and of itself, is not synonymous with senility.* Granted, the older we get the more experiences we've had to sometimes forget about. Yet, that's natural and normal. I, too, have had many experiences in life that, when I'm reminded of them, I realize that I've completely forgotten about them and . . . I'm not eighty, I'm only fifty-five! When examining these instances that I'm reminded of, I realized that all of them happened during certain traumatic phases in my life and, it seems, the mind is sympathetically kind-hearted, it has a way of "softening" or "fogging" those particular memories that may cause the heart pain upon clear recall of them. Still, there's much that I don't recall about various other times in my life, and I find that the details are often more than a bit fuzzy for events experienced more than ten or twelve years ago.

But, you see, the human consciousness holds all we've ever experienced, all we've ever seen, heard, spoken, and done. However, all of those events are held in the deeper subconscious level of our minds and not in the forefront of one's conscious mind where events of "today" have so much more impact and precedence.

In the Alzheimer's patient, loss of this *current-time* cognizance becomes increasingly apparent and should, therefore, be a flashing neon light that warns of deeper problems for the patient, the patient's family, and, of course, for close friends and business associates.

Examples

One of our first glaring indicators of Mary Belle's diminished level of cognition was when, shortly after she came to live with us, we sat down at the kitchen table one late autumn evening to pass the time in an active game of Monopoly. The game began normally enough until, after forty-five minutes or so, Mary Belle began exhibiting visible signs of agitation. It was clear to us that she didn't like it one bit that she wasn't acquiring the better properties and seemed to be actually pouting about it, yet continued on playing with determination (this *childishness* being a typical behavioral element of the disease). After another thirty minutes or so had passed, she couldn't seem to differentiate the dice from the houses and hotels and, when her turn came to make her move, she'd grab the houses off the board and throw them instead of the dice. She was clearly confused. And, as quickly as we could, we let her "win" and put the game away.

As the weeks passed, we observed that she couldn't concentrate on any one task or game for more than a few minutes. Her attention span was extremely short-lived. She wasn't able to work the many puzzles we'd bought her, so we searched the stores for those containing 100 pieces or less. Finding these wasn't as easy as you may imagine, for the simpler puzzles had images geared for very young children and were not appropriate for an adult. Keeping the importance of maintaining her self-esteem in mind, we didn't want to bring her obviously *juvenile* activities to work on, for fear of making her think that we thought all she could manage were childish projects. I personally think that the puzzle manufacturers should recognize and address the growing number of elderly Alzheimer's people in society and perceive the need to create puzzles with 100 pieces or less that depict adult themes instead of cartoons, Disney characters, or perhaps offer easy-to-assemble scenic images. Eventually, we had to resort to searching for puzzles with not more than fifty pieces.

After we discovered that she couldn't manage the more common games and puzzles, we wracked our brains in an attempt to come up with more simplified activities to keep her mind exercised. This was important to us. We wanted to try to keep her mind stimulated, yet, also, didn't want to give her activities that were too difficult for her to perform and succeed at. This was not an easy task for us. This was a quest that appeared to have a fine line between the two polarized ends of it. We very much wanted to provide her with activities that made her feel a personal sense of worth and accomplishment.

In an attempt to provide this sense of self-fulfillment and accomplishment for her mother, Sally came up with what she thought was the perfect solution. She went up to her mother's bedroom and lugged down a large and heavy bank bag full of her deceased father's massive collection of old wheat pennies that Mary Belle had been saving for many years. I'd never seen so many pennies. In this canvas bag were coins inside plastic bags, coin tubes, envelopes, and even small jars. With extra exuberance purposely applied to her tone of voice, Sally then asked her mother if she would like to finish sorting the pennies by date (something her father had been doing while he'd been home dying of a brain tumor).

Mary Belle's eyes lit up like two Fourth of July sparklers. "Oh yes!" she piped up with excitement. "Rudy would like that."

But she kept mixing up the date piles that Sally had separated out on the kitchen table. She kept getting confused about the whole point of her project (that of separating the coins by dates). So then Sally made an attempt to simplify the task even further. She made dozens of paper tags with the dates written on them so her mother could easily differentiate the separate piles. Still she mixed them up and couldn't manage the activity with any measure of success. Not wishing to cause her mother further frustration (or embarrassment), Sally put the coins back in jars and they were quickly forgotten. The project idea was a failure.

We tried additional types of activities, each one more simple than the one preceding it. Yet nothing appeared to be manageable enough unless it was an activity such as sitting out on the deck staining scrap wooden boards, coloring in velvet pictures with paint pens, dusting, or washing the dinner dishes. I personally had a problem with her doing the dishes because that was a routine household job I normally did and didn't want Mary Belle's family and friends to think we had put her to work "doing our housework." I know that may sound silly and absolutely ridiculous to some readers; however, people's reactions to such simple and completely innocuous intentions can be quite amazingly contrary to the pure innocence that originally generated the activity. I didn't want people having misconceptions about her stay in our home—no matter how silly it seemed or no matter how someone could twist our good intentions. I'd seen it done more times than I'd like to admit to. It's sad and pitiful to see that kind of misperception in human thought and opinion, yet it happens all the time.

The next activity-related incident happened when Mary Belle saw me doing the weekly ironing in the kitchen. She wanted to do it and didn't mince words about expressing that desire. Again, I thought about the possible misunderstandings that could arise if she told friends that she was doing all of "our" ironing. How would that appear to those people who had no idea that we'd been searching so hard to provide Mary Belle with projects that she could accomplish with ease and make her feel good about herself—make her feel that she was a productive member of the family and helping with the household chores she wanted to do for us? Well, I put her off as long as I could, before she became so insistent that she actually began to physically push me away from the ironing board (this, unbeknownst to us, was the first sign of Alzheimer's aggression coming to the fore). Eventually I relented, rather than see her become so agitated, and we soon discovered that ironing was a dangerous activity for her to perform because she'd leave the appliance lying face-down on the board or on an article of clothing and, after becoming easily distracted by something else in the house, she'd walk away from it—leaving it on.

The next time I had to iron, she pushed me aside again. This time I just told her that, since she did it last time, it was my turn. We'd take turns. This appeared to appease her and she walked away without incident. When the pile of wrinkled laundry was again mounded high enough to tackle the chore of ironing, I took the iron and board down to the basement where I performed the task thereafter without her ever knowing I'd done it. Removing things from the sight also removes them from the mind and, by doing this, the caregiver soon learns to lessen the frequency of having to tell the patient "no" and, consequently, also circumvents potentially combative incidents that can so readily result from her being denied a single-minded "want-of-the-moment."

The first time I vacuumed, Mary Belle intently strode up to me and forcefully attempted to grab the handle out of my hands. This time, though, I had to be firm right from the outset. She was not going to vacuum. I was not going to let her do the daily household chore of vacuuming because she had bad knees and a heart condition. This chore involved physical exertion. This one element of work was definitely out of her league for valid health purposes and, through gentleness, I took the time to fully explain my reasons why she needed to leave this particular activity to me. I repeatedly stressed the aspect of what just a little physical exertion can do to one's heart at this elevation, and also added that I just plain enjoy doing the vacuuming because it gives me additional exercise. After I was finished voicing all of my reasoning, it was clearly evident that she didn't like being told that she couldn't do something but, fortunately for all concerned, she did seem to understand (and accept) the reasoning regarding this particular household job. When I saw her walk away in a dejected pout, I went to the kitchen drawer, pulled out a clean rag, and offered it to her. "Want to dust instead?" I suggested, hoping to perk her up. The pout vanished with the appearance of a broad smile of satisfaction as she took the rag and quickly busied herself about the house. Because she couldn't seem to remember where she found the items that she had just picked up and dusted off, few knickknacks were ever returned to the same place, yet that didn't matter a whit to me because she ended up gaining that all-important sense of being a productive person and achieving some sense of purpose in the way of "helping us out" by being an active participant in keeping her new home neat and clean. Dusting in exchange for vacuuming. Wasn't a bad deal. Wasn't a bad deal at all. It turned out to be a good trade-off that satisfied everyone and avoided a confrontation. It satisfied her need to feel useful and it satisfied our concerns over her performing activities that could possibly exacerbate her heart or knee conditions.

One evening, when Mary Belle and I were sitting together in the living room, she was comfortably seated in her new recliner, contentedly snacking on a bowl of macaroni and cheese that Sally had fixed her. She was watching television, and I was deep in concentration, reading some research material for one of my book projects. Suddenly, my thoughts were interrupted when I heard her talking in a conversational manner. Since we two were the only people in the room at the time, I naturally assumed that she'd been addressing me and that I'd been too engrossed in the reading material to notice or properly respond. I immediately felt a pang of guilt for behaving in such a rude manner—as though I'd been ignoring her—so I gave her my full attention. What I saw when I looked over at her didn't correspond to what I'd *thought* it would be. She wasn't talking to me at all. Instead, she had the bowl of macaroni up to her ear and was having a lively, imaginary *phone* conversation with it. As politely as possible, I nonchalantly informed her that the bowl of food was not a telephone. "Oh," was all she said, placing it back down on her lap to finish eating from it. End of event. She never appeared to feel embarrassment over her mistake. In fact, it seemed as though she forgot about it as soon as she began eating again.

Another night I'd stayed up writing until 3:30 in the morning and, instead of trudging up to bed and taking the risk of waking everyone up with the racket of the gate lock at the top of the stairs, I curled up on the living room love seat and quickly fell asleep. At 5:30 A.M. Mary Belle was standing before me, dressed, and bright-eyed, telling me, "I need some of that black stuff."

Huh? Whaaat? Black stuff? What black stuff? And, I thought through my fuzzy, half-awakened state, *how'd she get down here?*

Not having had more than a couple of hours' sleep, I wasn't exactly in the greatest mood to be awakened in such an unexpected manner. As the sleepy fog began to clear from my brain, I finally figured out that the "black stuff" she was talking about was coffee; so, in a semi-stupor, I shuffled my way into the dark kitchen and brewed a fresh pot for her before immediately returning to the much-desired couch to capture more dreamy winks.

Soon, she was standing before me again.

She poked my shoulder.

I opened an eye and looked at the knees of her slacks that were directly in my vision.

"How do . . . do I *get* some of that . . . that, oh you know, that . . . black stuff?" she asked.

Peering up at her through one half-opened lid, I naturally replied, "You pour it into a cup," just before shutting my eye again.

"Okay," I heard her say in a satisfied tone while walking away from me.

For the third time she stood before me. Poke. Jab, jab went her finger on my shoulder. "How do I get it *into* the . . . the glass?"

Opening that one eye again, I now saw that she stood before me holding a water glass.

Okaaay. It was evident that it was time for me to get up and get her a proper cup and fill it with coffee, because verbal directions weren't going to help her.

With that small task taken care of, she smiled back at me in complete satisfaction. "Thank you," she said, turning and walking over to her recliner with the intention of sitting and waiting until Sally and I were up for the day.

Sally slept on for several more hours because she'd also been up late working on metal sculpture in the basement workshop.

Me? I was up for the day. I was up, because, although I had tried to curl back up on the love seat and fall asleep again, every time I looked up to check on Mary Belle, to make sure she wasn't slipping out the back door, she was sitting in her chair staring at me. Having someone stare at you while you're trying to sleep is not particularly conducive to gaining that sleep.

The mystery of how Mary Belle had gotten downstairs in the first place was quickly solved when Sally came downstairs. She'd told me that she'd left the upstairs gate unlatched the night before when she went up to bed because I was still downstairs working.

This incident with the coffee was definitely not a rarity. In fact, it, and others much like it, were happening at an accelerated rate. More and more, we noticed that Mary Belle was forgetting how to do the simplest everyday things. Her ability to remember the processes involved with accomplishing some of the most common daily activities was declining at a rapid pace. When she did remember how to pour the coffee into a cup, she'd forget how to add her cream and sugar. It appeared that the addition of those two necessary ingredients to her coffee became far too complex for her to manage. Even when one of us took the instructional time to stand with her at the kitchen counter and moved the two containers right in front of her in an effort to help her become more self-sufficient, she couldn't seem to manage the activity. A simple process became a feat too great for her to manage by herself. She'd either take the spoon, fill it with sugar, and then empty it directly into the powdered creamer container instead of into her coffee, or she'd dump double doses of sugar into the awaiting cup of coffee and completely forget about adding the creamer. Once, she even poured the coffee directly into the sugar bowl instead of into her empty cup. I can't tell you how many times we've had to toss out both containers' contents because they'd been mixed together. Sally made a valiant attempt to get her mother to go back to drinking her coffee black as she'd done all her life but, more recently, Judy had gotten her accustomed to adding the cream and sugar. No amount of cajoling could alter that newly gained habit. Coffee was no longer a palatable drink to her without the addition of lots (and lots) of sugar and cream. We eventually relented. It wasn't that important to make a fuss over, and it was just so much easier for either Sally or me to prepare the coffee for her. Issues like this are soon sorted out by the discerning caregiver. Every day is a learning experience—especially for the caregiver.

The frequency of the times when Sally's mother would suddenly ask with great animated indignation, "Is there a *bathroom* in this place?" increased. She'd forgotten where the bathrooms were, and, what was even more surprising for us to realize, was the added fact that she also didn't readily recognize a bathroom when she was already standing directly in front of its door. Or else we'd often hear her ask one of us, "Are you two going to spend the night here? If you are, you can sleep in my room until you need to leave for home." Clearly, statements such as these were generated from her believing that we were merely visiting her at her townhouse and we needed a place to sleep while we were there. Such statements obviously showed us that she had no cognizance as to "place." She just didn't know where she was, a good deal of the time. Therefore, we'd have to often keep reminding her that this was our home, that she was living here with us, and that we wouldn't be "leaving" any time soon.

There were other times when Mary Belle would state that she was going into the kitchen for a glass of water, and then she'd return with a fork in her hand instead of the desired glass of water she'd intended to get. Or, if she did manage to successfully get that glass of water, the faucet would be left running full blast without her remembering to turn it off, or the glass might be filled with hot water instead of cold.

The concept of "gender" no longer held any type of significant differentiation for Mary Belle's new worldview. To her, everyone was a "he." And it did no good to keep reminding her that "there are no he's in this house except for the cordon blue finch." Didn't matter, everyone was a he. She couldn't recall her age, couldn't tell you what state she was residing in, what month it was, or who she just talked to on the phone. Nine times out of ten, she would even deny that

63

she'd had a phone conversation, even if she just finished hanging up the receiver. Then you were called a liar for trying to remind her that she'd just finished talking to her sister.

As mentioned earlier, writing her own name had become an impossibility unless we wrote it out on a piece of paper for her to copy from. She confused her children's names and began calling her son "that man." Her attempts at following a conversation were not successful, yet she would make an attempt to participate, only to come up with totally unrelated, disconnected statements or complete nonsense.

The cognitive verbal skills were either completely lost or tangled, whereby the words emitted were those associative terms connected to the mental thought rather than those precise terms directly related to that specific thought. For example, around the time of Halloween when she recognized signs of the holiday after I hung Indian corn on the door and placed gourds on the dining table, she'd say, "orange thing" for pumpkin, or "ghost" instead of Halloween. Understanding Mary Belle's attempts at conversation became an exercise of associative wordplay and we grew expert at deciphering her uniquely individualized manner of speaking. Although she may have had the correct word in her head, verbalizing that word was becoming beyond her capability; therefore, descriptive terms or associative words would be voiced instead, and we'd have to connect the spoken word(s) to her intended meaning. It was like learning to decipher audible code.

This initial stage of Alzheimer's is perhaps the most difficult for the patient, because she still has enough mental awareness to recognize the diminishing ability to remember and speak clear thoughts. The patient gets extremely frustrated over not being able to verbalize thoughts and perform the simplest common tasks anymore. Because of this recognition, it's extremely important for family members, friends, and the caregivers to show patience and convey attitudes of understanding. Sometimes Mary Belle would get so frustrated with herself while trying to verbalize her thoughts to us that she'd throw up her hands in absolute disgust with herself, saying, "I'm just so stupid, I'll talk . . . talk to you . . . you some other . . . time . . . year!" and then walk away in complete exasperation. We'd tell her that was okay and that her inability was just due to the disease. Over and over, we took the time to reassure her that she was not stupid. Sometimes when she spoke nonsense and she realized it, we'd all smile and then make a joke out of it. Humor can play an important role in helping to deal with these types of incidents, both for the patient and for the caregiver.

Yet, more and more, as time progressed, we witnessed the decline in her verbal ability. When she tried to say something, it rarely made any sense because she totally mixed separate thoughts together in one sentence; more often, though, these thoughts came out in disconnected phrases rather than whole sentences. She may have come up to one of us with an attitude expressing extreme urgency and say something like, "When . . . when are those . . . men coming . . . with the . . . oh, the . . . *spoons!*"

And, naturally, we'd respond with, "What men, Mary Belle? What spoons?"

"What men?" she'd reply. "Men where? What spoons?" Then she'd walk off shaking her head as though she had never had anything of importance to tell or ask us. This was because her original thought had been completely forgotten.

This example was not unusual. During the course of a single day, Mary Belle began dozens of "important" statements and "urgent" questions, only to end up making you sound like the person who didn't know what you were talking about. This, of course, also represented a day filled with continual interruptions for the caregiver or family members. You would stop what you were doing and try very hard to be patient with her while she struggled to get her words out. Then, when she did, it didn't make any sense, and you had to try to pick the statement apart to find logic in her intent.

Most times, there was no rationale and the situation was resolved by her just walking away from you and then forgetting that the entire incident had happened. If this occurred while I was writing a book on the computer, and in the middle of a carefully worded philosophical thought, it was extremely frustrating. Yet, patience and understanding are the operative words. You must always remember the basic fact that this individual has a disease that affects the mental processes and that she isn't intentionally interrupting you to antagonize you. She came to you with a truly urgent thought that she needed to quickly express and then forgot what it was, after not being able to verbalize it properly. Interruptions and nonsense become a normal part of a caregiver's daily life. Accepting those events goes a long way to lessening the stress of dealing with them.

Oftentimes, it's helpful for the caregiver or family members to take a time-out—to place themselves in the patient's position. Take time to think about it. How would you feel if you couldn't adequately verbalize the specific words to convey your thought? Or how irritated with yourself would you become if your words came out so jumbled that nobody could make heads or tails of what you were trying to say to them? You'd want people, especially those you love, to have patience with you. You wouldn't mean to be difficult or cause them irritation because you would be trying really hard to communicate with them. For the patient's caregiver, family, and friends, perpetual patience is the key reaction to this type of impaired communication and forgetfulness. Having patience with the impaired communication, and applying creativity in dealing with the loss of ability to perform simple activities, makes all the difference in how these new difficulties are managed and dealt with.

As caregivers, you want to make the patient feel as useful and as productive as possible. The last thing these people need to feel is worthlessness, so devising clever alternatives is important to both patient and caregiver. Although Mary Belle wanted to help us with house projects and the daily cleaning chores, her heart condition, blood pressure, and weak knees narrowed the options considerably. We let her dust and sort out old catalogs. Due to her forgetfulness and physical condition, we couldn't allow her to iron, use the stove, chop onions (use knives or any other type of sharp utensil), vacuum, shovel snow, rake leaves, etc.—all the things she begged to help with and would become angry at us when told no. Yet we could and did invite her to help us collect kindling, dust, stain or paint scrap boards left over from our construction projects, sort pennies from nickels, color in the velvet paint sets, look through catalogs for gifts for upcoming family birthdays, etc. Some days she wanted to be doing something so much that, one day, I found her down in the dog yard picking up doo with her hands. When I caught her doing that, I was aghast and told her that we had special utensils for that and she shouldn't ever use her hands for that chore. After I guided her back into the house and helped her wash her hands, I returned to my gardening. Not two minutes later, she proudly exited the back door holding up her chosen "utensil" for the job—a *serving spoon* from the kitchen drawer! This showed that she tried, yet didn't have the cognizant rationale to come up with the correct tool (solution). Picking up the dog yard was not a sanctioned activity for her because too much bending was bad for her heart and knees. Besides, I just didn't feel comfortable or right about her doing that sort of job around the cabin. There were cleaner things she could do if she wanted to help out.

Then there were those days when Mary Belle had no desire to do anything at all other than just sit in her recliner in the living room and look out the picture window at the mountain valley and watch the wide variety of birds coming to the porch feeders. These listless days, we noticed, were increasing, and the lack of interest in any kind of activity made one wonder what she was thinking, sitting there for so long. Was she thinking anything? Was her mind blank? Seeing her sitting like that for so many hours made me feel guilty for being busy, yet when I went over to her and inquired if she'd like to do something, she merely shook her head. If we asked her if she'd like us to turn the television on in her room, she'd smile and say, "No, thank you." So you'd leave her to do what she wanted most to do and go about your day.

Acceptance. Acceptance of the Alzheimer's symptomatic behavior is the key to good management as a caregiver. Compromise, too.

Acceptance and Compromise are the two golden keys.

You soon discover that you're always in the position of walking along the fine, invisible line of choosing between the necessity of attending to your own daily chores and business affairs, and gauging the "place" the patient is currently within. Whether she wants to just sit and gaze out a window all day or she wants to help with your chores is something that continually alternates on a daily (sometimes hourly) basis.

The acutely aware caregiver remembers to always work within that ever-changing framework and, consequently, each day is never the same as the one preceding it. Each day was a new challenge, a new presentation of events which were solely contingent on whatever psychological "space" Mary Belle was in that day. That "space" was very important. It was the critical criterion that served as the caregiver's cue as to the specific type of psychological technique that was best to employ for optimum patient management. By this I mean that, by being on top of the situation—being continually perceptive of the patient's mental frame of mind—the caregiver could take that valuable cue and immediately know whether the patient was in the psychological "place" that required responsive handling through sternness, humor, extra expressions of companionship, distance (because she wants to be left alone), or any of the many other methods of interactions that can be utilized.

Some of the various reference books on Alzheimer's that we researched appeared to have the caregiver spending her/his entire day as the "patient entertainer," when that's not even a logical scenario when applied to real time and real life. It's especially not a rational concept when the patient resides in the caregiver's own home on a permanent basis. The reality of that situation is that certain activities need to be attended to at home: chores such as routine house cleaning, laundry, and yard work. The telephone needs to be answered and conversations engaged in. Pets need to be taken care of. Meals must be prepared and dishes washed. The mail needs to be picked up, checks for the bills written, the grocery shopping done, house repairs attended to, etc. And, if you're also self-employed as both Sally and I are, there must be time allotted to devote to that income-producing endeavor that pays the living expenses. Sally is an artist and a jeweler. She needs time to work down in the basement workshop to spend making the varied creations that the local shops sell for her. I'm a writer and require time to write and, depending on the type of book I'm currently working on, I need time to find the research books I need to order, and then time to study them.

An at-home caregiver still has a life full of personal aspects to attend to. None of these necessary elements vanish from one's life just because someone has come into the home who requires care; therefore, to imply that the home caregiver is a patient's constant "entertainer" is just ludicrous. It's terribly misleading for those who suddenly find themselves unexpectedly having to care for a loved one in their home. The idea will only result in leading the caregiver through untold hours of frustration and personal psychological conflict. It's just not logical. It's just not reality.

At-home caregiving is just that—giving routine care to the *patient's* needs and to those of *yourself* in your own home. The caregiver's full understanding and personal attitude toward this fact is what can turn each new day into a dreaded curse or a sunny blessing. The at-home caregivers are unique. They don't have the luxury of those nursing home workers who get paid to give care for the duration of an eight-hour shift and then leave it all behind when they walk out the door of the institution, drive away toward the privacy and peace of their own home, and do whatever they want to do for the rest of the day or evening. Nursing home workers have a personal, separate life away from their work and have the pleasurable advantage of getting away from the dementia for a time to enjoy physical and psychological respite and privacy. The at-home caregiver has no such opportunity to indulge in these luxuries, other than when an outside respite caregiver is paid to "spell" them for a few hours each week (or whenever there's the extra money available for such purposes). The Catch-22 here is that *you* are the one who has to *leave* your *own* home to get that small measure of this much-needed (and required) peaceful time. Yet this was enough. At least for Sally and me, it was enough. This, we found, is enough when love dwells within the caregivers' hearts.

Hoarding and Possessiveness

Those who are already familiar with the symptomatic behavioral characteristics of Alzheimer's will be quick to tell you that hoarding and possessiveness are commonly demonstrated basic traits of the disease. As with the "loss of cognition" characteristic, humanity on the whole can generally exhibit some measure of these two behavioral elements without actually having Alzheimer's. We all have lapses of memory. We all have some sense of ownership. And some of us even have a tendency to hoard (or we may prefer to call it "collecting") certain items for a wide variety of reasons. Yet in the Alzheimer's patient, these characteristics are greatly amplified.

Figuring out the rationale behind most of the particular items that an Alzheimer's patient chooses to hoard is usually not a difficult task for the caregiver, yet there are those items that can appear to defy reason, and no associative logic can be discovered. Oftentimes, the hoarding is generated by a deep-seated fear. Perhaps the patient went through the Depression and hides stashes of coins. That's one example of a logical connection to the action. Maybe the patient is fearful of not getting enough to eat and stashes food in her/his room. It is not hard to figure out the reasons for these chosen items, yet, there are those that are far more difficult to make connective associations with. Some of these would be items such as paper clips, spoons, little pieces of blank paper, a piece of cloth, etc. To the caregiver, these items don't appear to represent any logical reason for the necessity to hoard; therefore, the "why" of it is only found somewhere deep within the patient's own mind. And, if you inquire as to why they're so interested in collecting these particular items, they may not be able to tell you the reason or to adequately articulate the cause for such hoarding. They may, in fact, even deny that they're doing it and, when confronted with the piles of "stuff" as physical evidence, may give a wide-eyed look of surprise, turn to you, and ask, "How'd that get there?" This is a common Alzheimer's reaction that I call "turning the table." You may have been the one to initiate the question, but then it's batted right back in your own lap to answer.

Everyday people in society are known to hoard. I do too. I've known folks who hoard toilet paper for fear of the stores being bought out. I'm not quite that bad, because I seem to have a history of having favored items that, for whatever reason, eventually become unobtainable in the marketplace. I favor embroidered blouses. So when they come in style I have to stock up because they won't be back in vogue for maybe another four to six years and, during that interim, not one can be found. Same with my favored perfume scents that two manufacturers discontinued producing. Same with the lipstick I'd used for twenty years. Same with the brand and style of jeans I always wore. Therefore, whenever I discover something that I really like now, something that's really "me," I've learned from past experience to purchase it in quantity and store it away for future use—just in case. So from my example, I suppose you could say that I hoard certain items that become extremely rare to find in some years, but the Alzheimer's patient will hoard objects that have no particular or specific use (at least to the observer). It's not that he/she becomes some kind of pack rat whose room is littered with a wide variety of collected clutter; it's far more specific than that. Only certain items appear to be the central focus.

Possessiveness, at least a minuscule measure of it, appears to also be a naturally occurring behavioral trait coursing through human veins. We all have some sense of possession, whether it be of the non-material variety, such as that of a sense of accomplishment or achievement, in the way of having pride in the improvements we make on our homes, or an attained talent or skill; or whether it's of the touchable, material variety like a newly acquired antique, a piece of unique furniture, the spanking new SUV, whatever. Rarely can one truly say that they have absolutely nothing which they take a special pleasure in possessing or having personally achieved. This is natural and need not be indicative of a possessive or materialistic element of one's personality.

The sense of possessiveness in the Alzheimer's patient goes far beyond what can be considered as being the "normal" range, as exhibited by the general populace, for, frequently, his/her strong sense of ownership is attached to that which belongs to someone else. The patient often appears to display an emotionally intense and dramatic psychological retrogression to the stage of the two-year-old youngster who is continually shouting, *"mine!"* even if the item in question is *yours*.

When we first saw this uncharacteristic behavior in Mary Belle, we were taken by surprise and wondered about the *why*s of it. Instead of immediately overreacting to her claim to something of ours, we just walked away and privately discussed it. We considered the possibility that perhaps she'd been feeling some sense of loss. She could be fearing that she was not only losing her mental faculties, but also everything else in life and, therefore, there could exist an urgency to regain and retain what she'd left behind—using some form of convoluted thought process that was making her believe that she'd be regaining some of her personal things. Though our theories were nothing more than speculation into the possibilities of her newly displayed behavior, they sounded perfectly plausible.

Whether the patient is residing in a nursing home or living in the caregiver's home makes no difference. The rationale behind this fact is that the patient no longer has her own place anymore. She no longer has her own personal furniture surrounding her and that alone has robbed her of the old, comfortable familiarity she had of being in her own home. The use of her car has been taken away, so perhaps she feels some sense of loss associated with her former rights as an individual—the freedom to move about at will has vanished from her life. And perhaps only a few select items have been saved to treasure as her own.

Remember, Alzheimer's is a type of dementia whereby the patient's rational thought processes are continually declining at a rapid pace, a little more with each passing day. The mental feat of remembering which items within one's housing situation actually belong to the patient becomes increasingly difficult to successfully manage. Consequently, there appears to be a strong drive to maintain a stranglehold on one's personal possessions, even if it's perceived by others as possessiveness in the extreme.

Examples

When Mary Belle first came to live with us and we were unpacking her belongings, she gifted me with a unique religious article that I'd expressed admiration over. It was a Madonna and Child encased in a small wooden shrine that had little doors that opened. It was a small piece, maybe three by five inches, and I placed it on top of my rolltop desk. It sat there for perhaps three weeks until, one day while dusting, I noticed that it was missing. Sally, in putting away her mother's clean laundry in her dresser drawers, came across the item tucked back beneath the lingerie. When she asked her mother why it was hidden away, Mary Belle became indignant and exclaimed, "It's mine!"

Sally reminded her of the day she'd offered it to me. "But you gave it to Mary three weeks ago. You gave it to her as a gift."

"No, I didn't. You're lying. It's mine! She stole it from me!"

So the issue was dropped and none of us ever mentioned it again.

But there's a clue here to her behavior—a huge, glaring clue for the caregiver to pick up on. If Mary Belle actually believed that she never gifted the item to me, she would've had it out in plain sight in her room, instead of hiding it away so it wouldn't be seen—so maybe we wouldn't discover that she'd taken it back. The fact that she'd hidden it implied that she knew she shouldn't have taken it back. Or, you could also posit that she hid it so nobody would steal it from her again.

With this particular disease, there are unlimited possibilities for the caregiver to analyze. Was it plain meanness or spite to take the gift back and then flatly deny having given it in the first place? No, we didn't think that was the case. Was it merely a matter of forgetfulness? Probably. Did Mary Belle think I stole the item from her? A good possibility. Having lived with an Alzheimer's patient for over three and a half years, we now know that all of the above answers were plausible ones.

So, what did this singular incident teach the caregiver? It gave clear indication that it was not a wise move to accept a gift (of a personal possession) from the patient, to always decline the offer with graciousness by responding with something like, "Oh, no, Mary Belle, that's yours. I wouldn't dream of taking something that's so important to you. That was a really nice thought, but thanks anyway." Every single day that the caregiver learns something like that serves to make the job that much easier. In this case, the caregivers had learned that the patient's generosity can quickly turn to resentfulness and suspicion. The caregivers learned that it's more common than not for the patient to sincerely give something of hers as a gift and then take it back with claims that it was actually stolen from her. This behavioral element is quickly nipped in the bud when the caregiver kindly declines the gift in the first place.

Possessiveness of the patient's own things is understandable, due to the simple fact that the individual frequently has few personal possessions left at this point. However, possessiveness of other people's things begins to show itself in a wide variety of ways.

Early on, when Sally and I were still able to safely be away from the house for a time, and Mary Belle was left alone, we'd return to begin finding that some of the household items had been disturbed—moved around—some missing altogether. Sally would search and ultimately find them somewhere in her mother's room—hidden in a drawer, down in the bottom of her laundry hamper beneath clothing, or in a shoebox at the back of the closet. When she was approached and questioned about these items, Mary Belle's mouth would drop open and she'd ask us how they got there. Well, that was the question Sally had in mind to ask, so she would.

"Mother, this is Mary's. Why is it in your hamper?"

"Well, I don't know. Did she put it there?"

"Of course not. How did it get there?"

"Well . . . I surely don't know. Are you accusing me of taking it?"

"Mom," Sally would attempt to explain, "there's only the three of us living in this house. If I didn't put it there and Mary didn't put it there, you had to have put it there."

Shaking her head. "Nope, not me. I sure didn't do it. Maybe that man did."

This last reference from Mary Belle was the beginning of her hallucinatory events.

So we retrieved the items from the hamper, shoebox, or drawer and walk away from the no-win situation.

I use a special herbal toothpaste and, when I would reach for it in the medicine cabinet and it wasn't there, I just went into Mary Belle's room and got it from her drawer without saying anything to her. The first time this happened, I asked her why my toothpaste was in her drawer. She said that she had no idea.

I pushed for a response. "Did you think it was yours?"

"I use Crest."

"But Crest isn't in your drawer, mine is."

She shrugged in a noncommittal manner. "Did *you* put it there so you can call me a *thief?*"

Sigh.

Around and around goes the nonsensical verbal merry-go-round so you quickly jump off and vow not to step up on it again. But eventually that vow falls by the wayside as, at some point in time, you're forced to ride it with another incident—another day or another hour—for some other reason.

More and more, the caregiver quickly learns that many conversations are of the "no-win" variety and, consequently, wisely discovers that it's so much easier to simply walk away from them and, most importantly, *forget* about them. Yes, it can be incredibly frustrating. Yes, it's tiring. But you're dealing with someone who isn't thinking clearly or rationally. It's important to always . . . *always* remember that.

On one sunny spring day I was outside in the new garden busily planting flats of perennials that we'd brought back from the nursery. Sally and one of our friends were busy building a potting shed on the deck. Inside, Mary Belle was occupied with a new puzzle Tony had recently sent her. Everyone was focused on their individual projects.

When I went into the house to get a drink and took note of what Mary Belle was doing, I saw that she was very intent on her own little project. She was crunching up old newspapers and stuffing them in a big cardboard box. My initial thought was that Sally had given her mother a project to do. Yet . . . the more I thought about it, the more something bothered me about it. I went out onto the deck and asked Sally if she'd given Mary Belle a special job to keep her busy and, when she said that she hadn't, I suggested that she'd better go see what Mary Belle was doing then.

I went over to our friend to see how the potting shed was coming along and began a conversation about it. Soon we heard raised voices coming from the living room and we looked at one another as if to ask, "Now what?" We entered the cabin to see what the commotion was all about.

Mary Belle had completely stripped our china hutch of my daughters' and friends' framed pictures, the incense sticks and burners, and fragile figurines. She'd been packing them away into the paper-stuffed box.

We could initially extract no rational explanation for why she'd been doing this. Even after Sally removed each item from the box and showed it to Mary Belle and said, "Look, this is Mary's. That's a framed photo of one of her daughters' wedding day. This is a photo of Mary's mother and grandpa. This is my figurine. Look, mother," she explained in growing frustration while unwrapping another item, "this is a special engraved wine glass that one of Mary's readers sent her."

Mary Belle made a lightning-speed motion to grab the glass. "That's mine!"

Sally was faster. As she whipped it out of her mother's reach, she said, "No, mother, it's not yours. It belongs to Mary." Sally held it up for her mother to see. "See, her name is etched in it. Is that your name? Is your name Summer Rain?"

Ignoring the evidence, Mary Belle just kept repeating, "That's mine! That's *mine!*"

Sally put the glass down and pulled out another item from the box. She unwrapped one of her favored cloisonné vases. Frustrated, she repeated, "This is mine."

Mary Belle made another angered grab for the vase. "You liar! That's mine! You give that over to me right now before I call the police on you!"

"No, mother," came the soft and surprisingly patient response, "this belongs to me. All of this stuff was either in or on top of our china cabinet. The china cabinet is not yours. So why were you packing up Mary's and my things?"

"Well . . . I thought they were all mine."

Sally replied, "Even if they were all yours, why were you packing them up? You're not going anywhere."

"I was going . . . going to give them to . . ."

"You were going to give all this away?"

Mary Belle nodded. "Going to send them to my daughter."

"I'm your daughter," Sally reminded.

"To my *daughter*—to Judy."

"Judy. Why were you going to send our things to Judy?"

"I don't remember now."

So then, all of the items were gently placed back in their respective places in or on the china hutch and the incident ended. What Sally and I didn't like about the event was how quickly Mary Belle could get into things she shouldn't. That realization hit home like a ton of bricks. She obviously had had the time to make her way down into the basement to get an empty box and bring it back up to pack. The basement is off limits to her because it's unfinished and there's no handrail on the stairway, plus there's a hole in the cement floor where the well pump is, and she could accidentally fall into it.

For us as full-time caregivers, this one incident was telling. It showed us that, even though we're at home with Mary Belle, we can never get too involved with projects for any length of time without taking regular breaks to check on her. Just being home with her isn't enough. We learned that we not only needed to be home, we needed to be home *and* always keep one eye on her. Our conscious *awareness* of her, and what she was doing at any given moment, was an ever-present necessity.

Another prime example of the disease's symptomatic possessiveness trait that we've experienced with Mary Belle was the fact that she never let us forget that the Nova parked beyond the garden gate was hers.

Shortly after Sally returned from Kansas City with her mother's Nova, Sally's own 1987 Corolla died. Since we didn't have the funds it would take to make the necessary repairs, she gifted it to one of her friends who's a mechanic and wanted to completely overhaul it for his daughter. So, then, the only real passenger vehicle we had to take Mary Belle out in was her Nova. She didn't do well in the old GMC pickup that bounced her around on our mountain dirt roads. And our rusty CJ-7 Jeep was even worse. It bounced people about like rocks in a polishing tumbler. Besides, Mary Belle didn't like to ride in either truck, because they had torn seats and no floor carpeting. They were also difficult for her to get in and out of because they were so much higher off the ground than her little Nova. Both Sally and I liked our two, rattle-trap trucks because they were the four-wheel-drive workhorses of our place; one vehicle was primarily used for plowing the deep winter's snow off the driveway and grading it in the summer after each hard rainfall had crisscrossed it with runoff ruts; the other brought her cut firewood out of the forest and was our "general hauling" vehicle. Although neither was dependable enough for us to use for any distance trips more than forty-five minutes' drive from the cabin, they still had plenty of local utility left in their creaky bones. For our secluded location, they were absolute necessities of life that we greatly appreciated having.

Because Mary Belle was on Social Security, we took over her car insurance and annual licensing expenses. After all, since we no longer had the Corolla, we figured that it was no big deal to just exchange one vehicle's expenses for another's.

Yet, as forgetful as an Alzheimer's patient can get, she always seemed to remember that that Nova was hers, because we would frequently hear comments like, "Are we going to take *my* car?" or "That's *my* car out there, you know." When she made statements like that, the emphasis was always placed on the "my" element. Her attitude about "her" car was generated from a seemingly "sour grapes" source, after she discovered that she'd lost the ability to drive it herself anymore. Although she'd tried to sneak out of the cabin and start the engine (we kept all of our vehicles' keys hanging in the ignitions until that incident happened), we had to reinforce our concern for the dangers she was placing herself and others in if she drove. Her doctor also backed us up on this the next time she saw him. She was not at all pleased over having lost this right to use her own vehicle.

There were three main reasons operating a vehicle by herself presented a clear danger. First, the roads around our cabin are not flat countryside roads, they're narrow two-lane ribbons snaking around the mountainsides in hairpin curves with steep drop-offs on one side. Some of these are surfaced with loose gravel rather than the smooth pavement she'd always been used to driving over. Second, she was now in an unfamiliar locale and didn't have a clue whether to turn right or left on the dirt road at the end of our drive. She didn't know which roads to take to get herself down into the town of Cripple Creek and going anywhere else would only get her lost in these hills, for there are dozens of back roads and old mining roads. Third, she's just not capable of operating a moving vehicle anymore. She confuses the accelerator and the brake pedals, completely forgets to use a turn signal, ignores road signs, and doesn't put the gear into park when she stops.

When the issue of her not driving anymore first arose, she'd get on the telephone with family members and friends saying, "*They* won't let me drive my car." To overhear her make comments like that made me think that she thought we were nothing more than a couple of bullies who were depriving her of her rights, yet the hard reality of the serious situation made the issue an imperative one. Finally, she resigned herself to the fact by saying things such as, "You *should* be paying for the Nova's insurance because it's *yours!*" and "That's *your* car, I can never drive it anymore, anyway." Although we made the insurance and licensing payments on it, we kept it titled in her name for two reasons. One, it was still hers. Two, she couldn't manage walking any distance from it after we'd taken her somewhere, so she still required the handicapped plates we could get for it. But once in awhile, we would still hear an under-the-breath comment, "Hope you know that that's *my* car."

We had numerous experiences with Mary Belle hoarding things in her room. These, for the most part, involved food that was secreted away. She would not, I repeat, would *not* get her own food. Though we reassured her time and time again that the kitchen and all the food in it were for her as much as they were for us, she'd only eat if either Sally or I prepared the meal and brought it to her. Also, she had a delusional idea (another disease symptom) that her dog, Molly, was starving. Well, anyone who knows how much I love animals (Sally loves them too) would think it ridiculous, even laughable, that we'd allow any pet in our home to starve—when, in truth, we go to the opposite extreme and splurge on their quality of food by purchasing the more expensive brand that's high in nutrients and without any additives or fatty meat ingredients. So, because of this delusional idea she had, she insisted that she needed to give Molly at least half of every meal she had. The problem with that was that when Sally took Molly to our vet for the annual checkup and shots, the vet strongly informed Sally that her mother's dog was considerably overweight and needed to lose at least ten pounds. Try telling that to Mary Belle. She didn't believe it. She thought we were out-and-out lying to her about it because "Molly is starving." Period. This statement was repeated to whomever she spoke to on the phone. This statement was believed by some of the listeners.

So then, every time Mary Belle ate, we'd have to remind her what the vet said and tell her to stop giving her dinner to her dog. She'd get so upset with us that she'd get up from the table and take her full plate to the counter, then walk away without eating. All because she couldn't give half to Molly. Her reasoning was that "if Molly doesn't get to eat, then neither do I."

"Mother," Sally would urge, "please come back and finish your dinner, you've hardly touched a thing."

"If I can't feed it to my starving dog, then I'm not eating it either," came the usual reply.

Again, we'd go through the whole story about how the vet reprimanded Sally over the "fat" schnauzer, how Mary Belle was doing harm to her dog's heart by continually feeding her own meals to it. But Mary Belle flatly refused to believe either of us and would not eat her meal after being reprimanded for handing Molly food from her plate. She'd walk away with tears in her eyes, because she was truly convinced that *we were* forcing *her* to starve her dog. Yet even though every time Molly was at the dog food bowl (which we kept full all day long), I informed Mary Belle of the fact that she needed to *notice* that her dog was eating, she continued to maintain that the animal was starving. Even seeing her dog eat from the bowl of dry food did nothing to convince her otherwise.

Hence the hoarding of food in her room. In her lingerie drawers there'd be a food stash. If the rolltop was pulled down on her desk, that was an obvious indication that there was some food hidden underneath. Her clothes closet held a wide range of hiding places for her food caches, including the clothing pockets. Food could be found just about anywhere, even behind the television or under her recliner cushion.

Several times, while she was eating her meal, I caught Mary Belle sneaking chunks of food into the pocket of her slacks. These were not tiny morsels, nor were they the types of food that do well in clothing pockets. These chunks would be anything—a fat slice of juicy pork roast, half a piece of gooey pizza, mashed potatoes, or maybe even a square of freshly baked, freshly frosted bundt cake. When I did her laundry I learned from experience to check all her pockets for the forgotten food stashes—what a mess that could be if I didn't catch myself before starting the load.

After discovering the type of hoarding she did, we had to remind her that this was the mountains and that we needed to give great care toward not leaving scraps of food around or crumbs on the kitchen counter or floor. We kept cautioning her that she was going to draw field mice to her room if she kept hiding food all around it. We used that reasoning instead of addressing or going near the issue of her dog being too fat. We didn't want to go there because we knew from past experience that it did absolutely no good. This alternate rationale would stick for a little while and then, while cleaning her room or putting away her freshly laundered clothes, we would find new stashes of goodies or old ones we'd previously missed (some no longer palatable to man or beast).

What the caregiver quickly learns from this kind of situation is to work within (or around) the problem. You go into her room every couple of days (while she's downstairs) and quietly check out her drawers, desk, hamper, shoe boxes, etc., for perishable foodstuffs. Then, quite discreetly, you dispose of them. More times than not, she won't even know they're missing, because she'll have forgotten she hid them in the first place.

Being forced to nose around in Mary Belle's room didn't initially set well with me. I was brought up to respect other people's possessions, space, and privacy. I taught my own children the same respect for other people's space. Having to peek here and there about another person's room, and quietly open drawers without her hearing, made me extremely uncomfortable. The act was behavior counter to my conscience and I felt guilty as all get out for doing it. It made me feel like a common thief, a sneak (I'll be addressing the caregivers' false guilt in a later chapter). However it was a necessary chore in good and conscientious caregiving. Once I realized that fact, I was okay with it and accepted the secret activity as just another facet of maintaining household cleanliness, and one more aspect of learning to be a conscientious Alzheimer's caregiver.

The twenty-four-hour, at-home caregiver has many personal attitude adjustments to make—some attitudes to overcome. The feeling of guilt over going through another's belongings is just one of them . . . one of the easier ones.

Loss of Social Graces and Basic Living Skills

Unlike the two former symptoms, the loss of social graces and living skills is not a subtle, hard-to-miss indicator of this disease. When an individual eventually loses the ability to perform simple living tasks and begins displaying an increasingly uncharacteristic lack of respect for others through a behavioral tendency to toss basic manners and common courtesy to the wind, this person is most likely exhibiting the deepening stage of Alzheimer's, whereby one's normal attention to self-esteem and "politically correct" social behavior wanes like the phase of a darkening moon.

It is this stage which precipitates the dreaded time of decision for family members, because it has become apparent that the individual can no longer be trusted to be self-sufficient. The appearance of this stage marks the time when family members must face the hard facts and, in a mature manner, decide what type of new living arrangement will best provide the patient with the most healthful, safe, and psychologically secure environment.

This is the stage when familial denial does the most harm to the decision-making process. This is the stage that, depending on the family's level of acceptance of reality, can break or bond that family as a unit. All options must be carefully considered. As seen with our personal example which Sally outlined in the *Background History* chapter, there will usually be no perfect solution and concessions will have to be given to compromises.

Many times, cost will be the singular determining factor in making this decision, for assisted care facilities can range from semi-independent living apartments to full-scale nursing homes—all extremely expensive. Most elderly people living solely on Social Security cannot afford these types of arrangements, as they range, on the average, from $2,500 to $4,000 per month. Looking at an annual basis, one's savings, investment income, and retirement would not sustain this living arrangement for more than a few years at the most. So instead of searching for the *immediate* solution for one's parent, the family needs to expand the scope of their problem-solving endeavor and look down the road with an eye to the *long term*. The family has to keep in mind that, although the parent has Alzheimer's and the end stage is a terminal one, the elder can still live for many years. It is this fact that needs to be a main element when factoring in all aspects of the dilemma the family faces, because they will naturally want those remaining years to be ones of quality and enjoyment.

Most of the so-called "assisted living" facilities are, in truth, *minimal* assistance providers, in that the resident will not be monitored in such a way as to insure that the proper medications are being taken or that the resident is indeed eating well. These two factors are critical for the maintenance of wellness and for the prevention of emergency situations that could arise by way of a possible accidental medication overdose or the onset of malnutrition.

In our own research into the option of nursing homes and the assisted care facilities, we'd discovered that there are a large proportion of them that will not accept a resident who "wanders" or has been diagnosed with Alzheimer's. When we initially looked into respite care for Mary Belle, we considered the option of dropping her off at our local nursing home, which provides this type of care so that the at-home caregiver can attend to errands or merely get a few hours of relief. Yet, when we inquired about this service, we were told that they absolutely did not accept any visiting patient under their Respite Care Program who has ever exhibited the tendency to wander. This is because the institution doesn't have the additional personnel to manage a one-on-one observance of the visiting patient. In other words, they can provide a safe environment for an individual who will voluntarily remain within the confines of the building property, and occupy his/her time with activities, but they cannot provide the "sitting" service necessary for those individuals who tend to get it in their heads to suddenly walk out a door.

Being cared for by loved ones will most often be the first choice for one's parent, yet family situations of the adult children are wildly diverse and complex. Some have young families of their own, some have busy professional careers, some live in another state, some have jobs requiring travel, and others may not be able to afford a professional caregiver to come into the home while they're at work (this expense starts at $10/hr., and can go as high as $35/hr., depending on the rates of the individual professional as based on the level of care required for a specific patient's needs). The adult children's living situations can widely vary and reaching a satisfying solution that's agreeable to all parties involved is, more times than not, a difficult exercise in facing reality and reaching mature decisions. Yet, it must be done. It must be done because the parent can no longer care for herself. The parent is in a life situation that is compromising her safety and well-being—she can no longer cook for herself or attend to the most simple personal hygiene practices. A parent cannot be left unsupervised, to starve when she doesn't eat due to forgetfulness, or to be harmed when she mixes up medication.

We've noticed that the loss of living skills and social graces makes the patient appear childlike. The small boy who fights taking his bath, the little girl who hates having her hair brushed, and the pouting that goes on when told it's time to brush one's teeth, etc., are common responses. This stage of the disease evinces many behavioral characteristics of a three-year-old who never gives a thought to personal cleanliness or social mores. The child who impolitely stares at a disabled person or picks his/her nose in public is likened to the Alzheimer's patient who has lost regard for the usual common courtesies during this progressive stage of the disease. All generally accepted elements of social politeness that were formerly subscribed to by the patient (who once respected self and others), are suddenly absent as they revert to those of a small child who couldn't care less about such societal expectations and polite behavior. The respect for another's privacy is gone, thoughts toward self-respect are at an all-time low, no care is given to withholding hurtful or mean-spirited comments, personal hygiene is not a priority any more and is, in fact, perceived more as a task to be avoided at all costs.

When the patient reaches this stage of the disease, the caregiver manages best when having the understanding that she/he is actually interacting with an adult having the mind of a young child. This holds true for both the behavioral symptoms of having lost the social graces and the lack of living skills. A three-year-old cannot fix his/her own dinner or take medication. A young child this age gives no thought to, nor has any embarrassment over, picking his/her nose in public or saying the first thing that comes to mind to someone, even if that "first thing" is, socially, highly unacceptable or just plain rude. The caregiver responses to these incidents are adjusted accordingly.

When the patient picks his or her nose in public, the caregiver's response is not the same as the response of the mother of the young child who may quickly swat at the offending little hand and be stern in her reprimand. Instead, the caregiver may say, "Would you like a Kleenex?" or else the caregiver provides one and discreetly hands it to the patient.

Caregiver response to the childish behavior of the adult Alzheimer's patient needs to be appropriate out of respect for the elder's age. Although that adult may show incredibly childish mannerisms and characteristics, that individual is still an adult and, as such, is entitled to corresponding responses. Make no mistake that, for the caregiver, continually keeping this in mind is not always a knee-jerk reaction, for the natural initial response is to say something more like, "Oh, for heaven's sake, will you *please* stop picking your nose!" But, it's important to realize that the specific type of caregiver response will oftentimes elicit a like reaction from the patient. Calm and respectful win hands down every time . . . well, almost every time.

Examples

Most activities that normal people feel inclined to reserve for performing in privacy will be done in public by the Alzheimer's patient. The first time I caught Mary Belle picking her nose and wiping it on the furniture was when we were in the living room watching television. I was so shocked to see her perform this highly unsociable behavior in front of me that I didn't say anything to her for fear of embarrassing her (but soon discovered that she could no longer be embarrassed).

Unsure of how I should respond after observing her do it again, I told Sally about it in hopes of receiving an appropriate way to handle the situation. She suggested that I should just go ahead and tell Mary Belle to "stop picking your nose." When the opportunity soon arose once more, I couldn't bring myself to say that because, to me, it sounded rude and disrespectful. So, instead, I nonchalantly placed a box of tissue beside her chair for the next time it happened. That evening I had the opportunity to gently say, "Mary Belle, there's a box of tissues on the table beside you." Well, obviously I hadn't worded it quite right because she just looked down at the box and continued with her impolite activity.

I persisted and tried rephrasing. "Mary Belle, do you need a tissue?"

She said she didn't and went right on digging.

Now what?

So the next time I caught her at it I said, "You need to use a tissue for that."

And she reached for one.

Yes! Finding the right wording for a response to a behavior is one of the many puzzles the caregiver must experiment with and solve.

It appears that fussing with one's body becomes a common behavioral activity for these patients. Mary Belle would frequently have her fingers deep in her ears, up her nose, in her mouth, on her scalp, or rubbing on her toes. She's put scabs in her ears with her fingernails and Sally has had to treat them, but the nose seems to be a particularly strong attraction that's difficult to avoid giving attention to.

At 6:00 one morning, Mary Belle was in the upstairs hallway trying to wake us up with very weak cries. "Please help me. I'm dying." I'd been up late writing the previous night and was asleep downstairs on the couch. Sally was dead to the world up in the bedroom, yet was able to reach her mother before I did because there was a locked stairway gate barring my immediate access to the top of the stairs.

"Oh, my god, Mother!" I heard Sally exclaim.

When I finally gained the top of the stairs, my first thought was that the place looked like a crime scene. Mary Belle had picked her nose upon awakening, and it had been profusely bleeding. There was blood all over the bathroom floor tiles (she'd been shuffling around through it). Blood was splattered on the oak cabinets. The bathroom sink was full of blood-soaked tissues. A full roll of toilet paper, completely saturated as she'd been holding it up to her face and using it as a sponge, was sitting on the counter. The front of her nightie was covered as well as her gray bedroom carpet. The bed itself was equally a mess.

Not bothering to waste time asking her mother why she didn't get us up sooner, Sally put Mary Belle in bed and, by pinching her nose for a time, got the bleeding to subside. Then, while my friend was cleaning up the bathroom (she refused to let me help) Mary Belle got up out of bed and the blood began flowing again.

Because Mary Belle kept insisting on getting up, our efforts to control the bleeding were greatly hampered. She was frightened and, consequently, quite combative. She kept pushing our hands away. Our efforts were futile and Sally had no recourse other than to finally call for an ambulance which took her mother to the emergency medical center in Woodland Park. There the doctor cauterized and packed the nostrils. Once home, Mary Belle could not keep her hands off the packing, so Sally had to affix medical tape over the nose to protect the packing from being pulled out.

We tried to get Mary Belle out of the house and give her some social contact once in awhile, yet, when in public, there was no telling what she might do. One time, when Sally treated her mother to a nice dinner out at one of the better casino restaurants in town, Mary Belle stared so hard and long at another diner that Sally became increasingly embarrassed. Staring at others in public is a common trait for Alzheimer's patients. They may not even realize that they're doing it, yet it becomes unnerving for other people and, many times, their reactions are not generated from a position of complete understanding.

At home, too, Mary Belle tended to stare. When I tried for a little leisure respite time with a good book, it was extremely difficult to obtain that relaxed leisurely "mood" when someone was staring a hole through me while I was reading. So I'd take the book to the chaise lawn chair we put in the basement for the express purpose of getting some relief from having eyes constantly on us. The experience could be quite frustrating and unnerving. Privacy for the at-home Alzheimer's caregiver is harder and harder to come by as it becomes a rarity in one's life.

Privacy. The patient doesn't seem to particularly want any, so, naturally, there is no thought given to why anyone else living in the home should want any either.

As a child I was raised with respect for the privacy of other family members. When I became a mother, I, in turn, taught my children to respect the personal space of others. Nobody went into another's bedroom if the door was closed. And, for many years, we had a total of seven people (extended family) living in our home. Every one of them could expect and rely on obtaining their individual measure of privacy; no one ever felt a need to lock the bathroom door when they were in there. I'm sure Sally was raised the same way. Yet, having Mary Belle in our home meant locking that bathroom door because, when she saw a closed door, she perceived it as a door to open.

Once when I was in the bathroom at three in the morning, Mary Belle began opening the door. I reached to shut it and turn the lock while quietly informing her that I'd be right out. She left, only to immediately return with a pencil to use as a tool to pick the lock. Hearing her feeble attempt to gain access, I repeated my former statement. The next thing I heard beyond the door was water splashing on the hallway carpet. As sleepy as I was, I knew that that sound could only be one thing. I pulled the door open and found her squatting. She'd urinated right where she was.

"Mary Belle!" I said. "What're you doing? I told you I'd be right out."

"I'm going to the bathroom," came the nonchalant reply.

Hearing the commotion in the hallway, Sally awoke and rushed out. "Mother! What's going on?"

"Just going to the bathroom, is all," she replied very matter-of-factly.

Sally washed her mother up, put her in a fresh nightgown, and cleaned the carpet as best she could. The next day I took the steam cleaner to it. It was the first incident that marked the necessity of keeping the carpet steam cleaner handy.

Another incident also happened in the early hours of the morning. Around 2:30 A.M., we were awakened by a loud thump from the bathroom. Sally rushed in to find Mary Belle wedged down on the floor between the bathtub and toilet. Her underwear was down around her ankles and she'd urinated where she landed. Sally got her up and asked what happened.

Not even realizing that she was on the floor, Mary Belle replied, "I went to the bathroom."

She'd missed aiming for the toilet seat and went down beside it. She had a bit of bruising on her backside, and, because her skin was so thin, there were bruises on her arms from Sally lifting her to an upright position. Again she was cleaned up and returned to bed.

Another such incident occurred early in the morning when we were again awakened by odd sounds coming from the bathroom. We'd discovered Mary Belle standing in front of the toilet with urine pouring down her legs. She'd left a trail from her bedside to the toilet.

These last two incidents were out-of-the-ordinary events. Formerly, she'd had no problems with making it into the bathroom during the night, except for the one time she didn't wait for me to exit the bathroom. She'd had no previous accidents, and we suspected that there was a specific reason for these last two. We put our heads together to figure out what was different about her routine that could account for the nighttime incontinence and greater mental confusion during that time. The answer was her sleeping medication. As a fluke, I discovered that the cause was the Ambien that she'd recently been taking.

Ambien was a common sleeping medication prescribed by her doctor in an attempt to reduce or resolve the incidents of her increasing nighttime agitation and wandering tendencies. After we'd been giving her one pill upon retiring, and she still wandered and was awake and dressed at 4:00

A.M., we called the doctor to see if it was okay to give her an additional half. After reviewing her chart, she said that we could, but cautioned us to give her no more than that.

Well, now, Mary Belle liked those pills so much that she began asking for them as early as seven o'clock in the evening. We'd tell her that she couldn't take them until she was actually *in bed* for the night. So then she'd restlessly pace the floor while waiting for bedtime to roll around.

One night, about a week after her two incidents with early morning urination accidents, I found myself tossing and turning in bed. I could not sleep. I was so physically tired from working on a cabin construction project the day before, but the mind was as busy as a spider spinning her web—the mind just wouldn't shut down. After trying for three hours, I finally got up, went downstairs to the medicine cabinet, and took one of Mary Belle's Ambien in hopes it would do the trick. I then sat on the couch with a book, waiting for the desired sense of drowsiness to wash over me. Before long the words of the text were blurring and the lines of type were shifting. This reaction didn't seem right to me. Shouldn't I just be getting sleepy? I closed the book, turned off the light and, like a drunk, made my way to the stairway. I could not climb the stairs without doing so on all fours. My coordination was not maintainable and perception was greatly skewed. I made it to bed, and, just before falling into a deep sleep, vowed to read up on Ambien in the morning.

The following day, I did just that. Ambien was a medication prescribed for insomnia and, as such, was a nervous system depressant. This was what was causing Mary Belle's nighttime loss of coordination, why she missed sitting on the toilet, why her mental confusion was greater during the night, and she had less bladder control making it to the bathroom during that time. I never took another Ambien, and neither did Mary Belle. Because she hadn't been on the medication for more than a few days, we were safe to withhold it without the possibility of her experiencing any withdrawal symptoms. But she fought hard to get us to give it to her at night. She wanted those sleeping pills so bad that she'd get angry and combative and try to push me out of the way when I barred her access to the medicine cabinet. Then she threatened to sneak down during the night to get them while we were asleep. But she couldn't do that because of the locked gate.

Every night for a week, we went through the same thing at bedtime. Mary Belle tried every means she could think of to get her pills from us. She tried tears (sympathy). She tried telling us that we were being mean and cruel to her (guilt). She tried hitting us (violence). She tried looking in the medicine cabinet for them, but we'd removed all medication beforehand (sneakiness). She even threatened to "get Grandpa's rifle and take care of everyone" (attempting to make us fear her). And then the Ambien was suddenly forgotten about. No more pre-bedtime combat over it, no more early-morning urinary accidents or missing the toilet. And no more night incoordination. Mary Belle was back on track.

For the caregiver, this experience became a golden lesson in knowing the necessity of the meds you're giving to the patient. I'm not advocating a personal experimentation with them as I did, because you're never supposed to take another person's prescribed medication, but do get out the *Physician's Desk Reference* (or other medication text) and take the time to educate yourself about each medication's possible side effects so you're not caught off-guard when one or more of them begin manifesting themselves. Know all the potential symptoms they're prescribed for, and be aware of the patient's behavioral/physical changes *after* ingesting the new drug. I'm not sure we would've associated Mary Belle's nighttime mental confusion and incoordination with the medication if I hadn't personally happened to sample one of her tiny Ambien pills. Please, learn from my own experiment.

The issue of privacy was touched upon earlier. Privacy is one of many luxuries of home life that few folks think to count as one of their many blessings. Yet, for the at-home Alzheimer's caregiver, privacy is not a given.

Mary Belle went through our desks whenever we were otherwise preoccupied with projects that took our attention away from her for any length of time. Once I overheard her telephone conversation when she was telling her sister the amount of one of my royalty checks. That really upset me, because that's nobody's business but mine and Sally's. Mary Belle had seen my check attached to a deposit ticket that we were about to take to the bank and the amount was forever after engraved on her mind. She clearly felt no compunction about sharing that figure with others. What she didn't realize was that I only get paid every three months, and, out of each check, Uncle Sam demands a gluttonous portion in my four estimated tax payments through the year. She had no idea of what our finances *really* were. Think about how attractive the amount of your own employment check would look like if you only received one four times a year. That's what Mary Belle saw, and so she believed that that was a *weekly* check and, therefore, "We have lots and *lots* of money!" So she believed—so she told everyone she talked to. And it did get irritating that we had absolutely no privacy in this matter and people got the wrong impression from hearing her many convoluted and delusional statements made about our private affairs.

Personal hygiene is another issue we had to constantly stay on top of. Normally, one isn't used to keeping track of how regularly another person brushes his/her teeth, and isn't responsible for knowing how routinely a shower is taken; but, with an Alzheimer's patient the caregiver has to be aware of someone else's schedule of normal hygiene care. I had to write down the days that Mary Belle took a shower on our household calendar, because she wouldn't believe us if we said that it was four days ago. The calendar became a necessity, because, in our busy schedule, we'd often forget and then realize that perhaps she hadn't taken one in nearly a week. We needed to keep closer tabs on it.

A shower for Mary Belle meant our involvement, because she'd do various unpredictable things like throw her clean underwear into the streaming water, or get in and fiddle with the controls and end up closing the drain and standing in a tub filled up to her knees with water, or move the temperature control and risk the possibility of burning herself. She might completely forget to wash her hair, exiting the bathroom with bone dry hair and then insist she washed it. She might not use soap. She might take a two-minute shower and claim that she was in there a long while, and no amount of arguing over it would convince her that she was not in there for a long time. So her bathing involved one of us making sure that she had the shower set right and didn't mess with the faucet settings. It involved making sure she used soap and actually washed her hair.

Caring for her teeth was something she'd never think to attend to if we weren't there to see that it was regularly done. She'd hide my herbal toothpaste in one of her bedroom drawers and then claim that she had no Crest when she'd hidden that somewhere else in the room (perhaps in a shoe box) and we had to hunt for it because she refused to use any other brand. We didn't play this hunting game for long. We kept a backup Crest in the linen closet where we could easily avoid the need for any future searching process. The caregiver quickly learns the tricks of the trade that serve as keys to making life so much easier.

Sally routinely gave her mother a pedicure and attended to her foot conditions (corns and the like). Mary Belle was also frequently seen fussing with her toes and, when Sally applied medicine to them, they then became an even stronger magnet which we had to continually tell her to leave alone while the solution was drying.

We had to remove the bathroom wastebaskets because Mary Belle began depositing her used toilet paper in them.

I've even found those in her bedroom wastebasket when I've gone in there to clean. I've found them collecting in the bathroom sink. I've found them in her clothing pockets when I've laundered her clothes. I've found them in her desk drawers.

The frequent incidents of unkind comments made by Mary Belle had to be accepted with the grace of understanding. This rudeness is a commonly recognized behavioral aspect of the disease connected to the loss of social graces and does take some getting used to. The familiar saying, "consider the source," never fit a situation more appropriately than with an Alzheimer's patient. Keeping this in mind at all times takes the poisonous sting out of potentially hurtful words and makes them less personal.

One day, when Sally was away on business, I took over her job of cooking (it's Sally's kitchen; she loves to cook and is excellent at it). For breakfast this day I fixed Mary Belle fresh orange juice and a Western omelet along with a side of O'Brien potatoes. For lunch I made her a grilled turkey and cheese sandwich with a fresh garden salad (chives and green onions picked from our garden). Both were appreciatively eaten when I delivered them to her lap in front of the television. At dinner time I made her spaghetti with Sally's delicious homemade garlic and olive Italian bread, set her hot meal on the dining table, added a wildflower to a vase, and called her to dinner. She walked in, took one look at the table, and turned on her heels.

"Mary Belle," I repeated, "your dinner's ready."

She reluctantly shuffled back in and stood beside the table looking disdainfully down at the steaming dinner. "I am not going to eat that," she whispered.

"Why not?" I asked in surprise. "You need to eat. What's wrong with it? I thought you loved Italian food."

"Well," she sarcastically harrumphed, "you just . . . just went and set that food down and . . . and expected me to come and eat it. Why is it out here on the table when you know I like to eat in the living room?"

"Because the spaghetti's got a lot of steaming sauce on it and I didn't want you to accidentally tip it onto your lap. Mary Belle," I tried to explain, "it's a lot safer and neater to eat this kind of meal at the table."

She gave me a glaring look, shook her head, and said, "Those flowers look like they're some kind of weeds."

My gaze shifted to the table vase. "Actually they are. Aren't they pretty together?" I asked while pointing each out to her. "See? These are purple fleabane, those are yellow ragwort, and the taller ones are fuchsia fireweed. They grow around the cabin and I thought they'd look pretty together on the dinner table. I just got done picking them."

Rather than commenting further about the wildflowers, she said, "I want breakfast."

"But you already had breakfast this morning. Remember? You ate a big Western omelet and fancy potatoes. You ate lunch, too."

In response, she just disgustedly sighed and shook her head at me.

"Mary Belle," I tried again, "look at the clock. It's seven in the evening and time for dinner. It's dinnertime now."

The head shaking continued as she released an over-dramatized sigh of exasperation.

"What?" I asked. "What's the matter?"

"I've known a lot of people in . . . in my life but . . . but *you* . . . you *really* take the cake. I've never known *anyone* like you!" And she walked away from the hot meal.

I was completely taken aback by what she'd said. I felt left in the dark as to what she'd meant by that last comment, so I followed her into the living room to find out. "What do you mean?"

"You just *plop* down my dinner . . . at the *table* no less, and then just *expect* me to come . . . come when you *call* as though I'm some little puppy dog! I've known a lot of people in my life, but," she repeated, "I have *never* known *anyone* like *you*! I'm *not* eating it."

Mmmm. There are those times when the caregiver forgets that the Alzheimer's patient has lost all sense of appreciation for what others do for them—lost their sense of politeness and social graces; therefore, because of this momentary oversight, my feelings were duly injured. So instead of simply dropping the whole issue (as I should have), I responded with my heart instead of with the mind's cool rationale under the circumstances.

"Mary Belle," I replied with open frustration, "you've never *known* anyone like me, because who do you know who has ever laundered your clothes and ironed them, fixed your meals and handed them to you on your lap in front of the TV, taken your dog to the vet's, treated you out to fancy dinners, changed your bed, cleaned up your room, helped you with showers, made sure you always get your medicine and . . ."

Since she knew that I was right and didn't want to openly admit to it, she quickly altered course and interrupted me with, "I know you'd just love to have . . . have me out of . . . of here. You and Sally hate me being here. I know you do."

Now, neither Sally nor I had ever given Mary Belle any reason for her to think or say that. Those same words were frequently used as her standard comment whenever Mary Belle realized that she wasn't going to win a verbal confrontation. I avoided her delusional statements and returned to the main issue at hand.

"Mary Belle, please, you and I both know that that's just not true so let's not go there again. You really need to eat. Please, go have your dinner before it gets cold. Sally and I spend good money on groceries and can't afford to keep wasting food like that."

She ignored me and defiantly strode over to her recliner and stubbornly sat down while the food remained on the table. It was a wonderful meal with homemade sauce and freshly baked bread. Wanting to give her plenty of time to change her mind about eating, I waited. I left her dinner out on the table for two full hours as I busied myself with other chores. She neither came to sit at the table to eat it nor took the plate to her chair. She was so determined to underscore her point regarding her displeasure over the dinner being set out on a table that she took it as far as not eating anything. I finally took the plate out onto the front porch and scraped the contents off into the raccoon bowl. Due to our patient's increasingly arrogant stubbornness, our four-legged forest neighbors were beginning to eat better than Mary Belle was.

This situational-specific behavioral aspect of the disease was especially infuriating to Sally and me, because, before Mary Belle came to live with us, we were light eaters whose grocery bill reflected that fact. Our bill was always a minimal one compared to most folks'. We weren't in the habit of preparing three meals a day, but rather each helped herself to something whenever she became hungry enough to feel like eating. Personally, I preferred to grab a piece of toast for breakfast and then not eat again until dinner time. Some days, especially if we'd been busy on house projects, we'd be perfectly content to merely snack on quick munchies like cheese slices or pieces of lunch meat rather than stop to prepare a full-blown meal.

Consequently, knowing Mary Belle would require three nourishing meals a day, we nearly tripled our grocery bills in order to provide her with a wider variety of three squares each day. Sally cooked wonderful meals including many not-so-common ones such as stuffed crab cakes, broiled shrimp and lobster, a variety of home-baked breads (sometimes baking three different flavors of loaves a day). So when this "refusing to eat a prepared meal" happened at least four times a week, we were deeply frustrated, because she alone was the reason we spent the extra money on our groceries in the first place. We couldn't stand seeing good food go to waste. Although no food really goes to "waste" around here due to all the wild forest critters we feed, we'd both much prefer it go into Mary Belle. We don't purchase roasts, lobster, and ground round for the foxes and raccoons. Their food is supposed to come from the feed store up the road.

Usually her reason for not touching the food on her plate was in direct protest for not being allowed to give half of her meal away to her overweight dog. The behavior was extremely childish and no amount of reasoning and reiterating what the vet said about the dog's physical condition would work. So, as caregivers, we tried to let the incidents pass without internalizing them by emotionally holding onto them. You're upset with the fact that good money for better-than-average quality of food was wasted. You're frustrated with the childish behavior. The incident makes you tend to have residual effects from the darkly frustrated mood. Yet, while you're doing that stewing, the patient will usually have completely forgotten the entire thing happened and proceed to happily act innocent of any impolite behavior. You're still mentally fretting over the irrational behavior and wasted food, while she's suddenly as happy as a lark after a spring rain. What's the point? The caregiver has to learn to not stew over things—to let them fall away like water running down a gold mining sluice. Stewing is definitely not good. It never serves any constructive purpose.

Understanding. Having the grace of understanding and giving consideration to "the source" is of utmost necessity for successfully dealing with the many variances of the Alzheimer's behavior that can oftentimes prove personally hurtful to the caregiver, who does so much and devotes an incredible amount of personal time to the patient and his/her needs.

What seems most hurtful are those off-handed comments not voiced to your face, but those that are of the back-stabbing variety you overhear being said to family and friends about you-the-caregiver, or about the living conditions, or regarding the quality of care the patient believes he/she is receiving. This "complaining" is a symptom covered in an upcoming chapter.

Nobody can healthfully live by themselves in a self-sufficient manner if they can't pour themselves a cup of coffee, can't safely and knowledgeably operate the simplest cooking appliances (such as a toaster), can't correctly dispense their own medication, correctly dial a telephone number, or recall how to write their name.

Many times Mary Belle stood in front of the kitchen faucet, but had forgotten how to get herself a glass of water. Those times when she did remember how to manage this task, she may have walked away, leaving the water running full blast or may not have moved the handle to cold to fill her glass.

She would never remember to take her medicine, brush her teeth, or take a shower.

She dressed inappropriately for the weather, often going out in the pouring rain, bitter cold, or blowing snow without any seeming awareness of weather conditions and the proper corresponding outerwear that those weather conditions require. She needed to be reminded that she wore a certain outfit more than two days in a row and needed to put on fresh clothing. She put her underwear on over her slacks, and, when dressing herself in the morning, frequently donned as many as seven layers of clothing at one time (usually multiple flannel shirts combined with full slips and knit undershirts).

She called 911 instead of dialing her sister's number.

She frequently went to bed for the night in her street clothes, shoes and all.

She talked to people on the phone and made all sorts of fabricated (delusional) statements that the listeners didn't realize were false. We'd find this out when we'd receive an angry call back from the individual or hear about it through the busy "family grapevine."

An example of this was when she told one of her sisters that "she wasn't being fed." The sister, naturally incensed over hearing this shocking revelation, immediately called Tony (Sally's brother) and told him to "get out to Colorado and take Mary Belle out of Sally's home because she's being starved!" Tony, being fully apprised of the ongoing situation after routinely talking to Sally several times a week and coming out to spend a week-long stay with us a couple of times a year, wasted no time in setting his aunt straight by informing her that his mother frequently flat-out *refused* to eat her prepared meals, for a wide variety of reasons.

What's so incredibly frustrating about this specific behavior was that the other people didn't realize that Mary Belle was saying things out of context or was making delusional statements off the top of her head, and, then these folks believed that you were being a terribly abusive caregiver by treating her badly or by being mean to her. This situation is, sadly, a common thread running throughout the experience of all at-home Alzheimer's caregivers. Though it would appear to be unfair and emotionally hurtful, that's the nature of the disease the caregiver must learn to contend with.

Another example of Mary Belle's mental confusion associated with the passing on of misinformation to those she talked with was when she told her daughter, Judy, that "Sally and Mary were building a *big addition* onto their cabin." Judy, curious as to how we could afford to do this, asked her mother where we got the money to build this big addition. Mary Belle then responded with a second delusion, "Oh, they have lots of money."

Well, if truth be told about this, the "big addition" was the little garden tool shed Sally and I were building ourselves (we have no garage). And the "lots of money" thing came from that one check she saw on my desk. With this incident, we didn't even bother calling Judy back to set her straight. The caregiver gets weary of always having to set people straight after the patient has made misleading statements. There are those times when you just opt for letting them ride.

The loss of social graces and the loss of living skills are two of the more obvious symptomatic behavioral elements that strongly point to probable Alzheimer's disease and are hard-to-miss markers, unless one is deep into choosing the self-protecting psychological escape route of denial.

Obsessive/Compulsiveness

Having the irresistible compulsion to perform the same actions over and over again, or obsessing over something, is not a psychological condition that's unique to Alzheimer's disease. Many people in society, individuals in all walks of life, exhibit these tendencies without having Alzheimer's. Some folks obsess over cleanliness and are driven by a compulsion to repeatedly wash their hands, or the kitchen faucet, or the toilet bowl. Some people obsess over the necessity of performing a specific routine and have the compulsion to never vary one step of that routine for fear something untoward will happen to them if they do. Others may be obsessed with a dire fear of the future, or of making a wrong decision, and have a compulsion to consult an intuitive reader regarding every move they make in life. These people have psychological behavioral disorders, but not necessarily the disease of Alzheimer's.

Those individuals who've been diagnosed with Alzheimer's frequently exhibit an associative symptom of obsessive/compulsiveness. This symptom is usually manifested by a newly acquired fear, a sense of extreme anxiety, or continual restlessness. Some patients will suddenly begin to pace and not know the reason why they're doing it. Some will feel the need to collect specific items. Others will repeatedly feel the need to check all the windows and door locks in a repetitive manner. This specific behavior is a desperate attempt to protect their physical well-being from harmful external dangers, and to also shield their emotional aspect of self from the possibility of experiencing upsetting events.

Because the Alzheimer's disease is a degeneration of brain cells, these obsessive/compulsive behaviors may be triggered by electrical brain currents stimulating some past and long-forgotten memory that the patient is unable to consciously associate with; however, subconsciously, there is some imprinted element connected with the past incident that incites and stimulates certain current time-responsive action related to those past events. Whether the patient can actually remember and be capable of identifying that particular past incident isn't germane to solving the "why" of his/her actions. All the individual knows is that he/she must keep repeating it in order to feel that all is right with the world. It's a bid to maintain a continuing emotional sense of security and an attempt to maintain it at a fairly undisturbed level of perceived acceptability.

Examples

When we first noticed that Mary Belle began asking the same questions over and over again during the day, we naturally attributed it to her increasing memory loss. We associated the repetitive questioning with her deepening forgetfulness because this symptom had been worsening by the week. She'd talk to someone on the telephone, and, when either Sally or I asked her how so-and-so was doing, she'd immediately give us a questioning look and say that "she didn't know because she hadn't talked to so-and-so in a long while." Yet she may have just finished talking to them less than five minutes ago.

Conversations and events that she'd participated in were quickly forgotten and, when we'd have occasion to remind her of them, she'd give us a look that conveyed she believed that we were lying about them. But, then, we'd notice that the type of repeated questions usually fell into a category that could be generally classified as being fear-based. She feared that her son wasn't actually going to come out to visit her as promised. Twenty times a day she'd ask, "when is Tony coming?" And, with patience, we'd tell her the day. We'd mark the day on the calendar so she could go check for herself, but then she'd forget that it was noted there and emphasized inside a big circle made with a red marker, and she'd keep asking her same question.

Mary Belle had a habit of examining our personal calendar. At first we felt as though this behavior was another affront to our privacy, but then realized that she was just fearful of missing a family member's birthday (everybody's being written down on the calendar and circled) so she felt she had to keep checking—just to be sure. When the caregiver expends the extra effort to determine the possible reasons behind the patient's repetitive actions, it can make life much easier.

Because the Alzheimer's patients most likely have been divested of a good portion of their personal possessions due to new living arrangements, the one remaining constant in their lives is that of family and friends. This, we determined, was the underlying reason why Mary Belle was daily observed carrying around her telephone list and continually obsessed with making notations on it after intently scrutinizing it for hours on end.

When she initially came to live with us, one of the first things Sally did for her mother was to get on the computer and update her mother's address book with enlarged type on 8 x 10 plain paper for easier readability. She stapled these pages together and put them on Mary Belle's rolltop in her room. This list, we soon discovered, was her way of feeling physically connected to family and friends. She would carry it about the house, keep it beside her living room recliner, write on it, and frequently hide it for safekeeping. Secreting this list away was her way of keeping these people "safe" and "unto herself"—private. When she forgot where she hid the list she'd deny hiding it and accuse us of stealing it from her. However, there've been times when it was hidden in the bottom of the kitchen wastebasket, and Sally would have to run her replacement copies because the former set had unknowingly gone out with the trash.

One of these replacement sets of her address list was covered with the penciled-in names of people she didn't know. She had marked in partial names with mixed-up addresses and phone numbers. These names were our own personal friends, family, and business contacts. Mary Belle had gotten into our Rolodex while we were out on errands one day and had copied down our personal list onto her own. When Sally discovered this, she asked her mother why she'd written down the names of people whom she didn't even know. Mary Belle didn't really know. She initially denied doing it. Then she said that some man did it. We concluded that the reason she did it was the possible rationale that her list was incomplete because ours had more names on it. So Sally would again run a fresh list for her mother. Usually, Mary Belle didn't believe that Sally did her list right and was obsessed with checking and rechecking it against our Rolodex. More penciled-in notations would be made again. And the entire process repeated. Every time Sally handed her a fresh copy of her address list, her mother would get on the phone with Judy and ask for names and addresses because . . . "Sally messed up her list and left everyone out."

Another example of this symptom was her obsession with bodily functions, especially with those of her dog. Imagine the family comfortably relaxing in the evening and everyone being deeply engrossed in a good movie—everyone but one individual who jumps up out of her chair and says the one thing that gets all six of our dogs barking and charging to the back door: "Let's go *outside* and go *potty!*"

Imagine that someone doing this not once during the movie, not twice, but five times in half an hour! It got real old real quick after the second time, because it turned into a confrontation, with us reminding Mary Belle that her dog was "just out" and her not believing us. She would actually push us aside if we tried to refuse letting those dogs out again. It got so bad that even the dogs were running for cover to hide from her obsessiveness. Poor Molly can only squeeze so much out of herself, and, if Mary Belle couldn't actually go outside and *watch* Molly relieve herself just to make sure, she'd insist that the animal never went . . . and "the poor thing *needs* to!" she'd insist, with tears of frustration brimming from her eyes. She then thought we were just the meanest people in the world for not letting her dog out.

If it was wet out from rain or snow, we'd show Mary Belle Molly's wet feet as proof that she "doesn't need to go back out because she just came in. See her wet feet?" This carried no weight toward resolution by rational thought, because then Mary Belle would claim that her dog stepped in her bowl of water and still needed to go outside. She'd claim this even if the dog had balls of snow stuck in her fur.

This was a difficult type of situation for both the patient and the caregiver. It's difficult because the patient truly believes the dog never went outside and is heartbroken that it will burst a bladder if we don't let it out. The patient cannot remember that the dog just came back in five minutes ago. The caregiver, on the other hand, is absolutely frustrated to tears from her own efforts to convince the patient that the dog did indeed go outside five minutes ago and that the caregiver is not being cruel to the dog. It's an impasse every time. The patient will not believe the caregiver, and the caregiver cannot convince the patient otherwise. Forget that movie, maybe you can catch it again late at night, when the patient's asleep, because you're now relegated to standing guard at the back door to keep her from trying to open it and physically go out with her dog. Her response can then be physically combative, or it can be tearful resignation that causes her to tell friends and family that "they're being mean to her dog. They never let her outside to go potty." The reason we held our ground on this one compulsive activity was that it was seriously affecting her dog, causing the animal to be neurotic. It's clear to see that Molly was totally confused over why she was being forced to go outside every five minutes. She started to visibly tremble when Mary Belle began this behavior. Molly plastered down her ears, cowered, and ran for cover beneath the nearest piece of furniture.

We did not allow our own dogs to go outside every time Mary Belle tried to sneak Molly outside. When I let our dogs out during the day and, held the back door open, I only let out those who ran past me. Those who didn't had made it obvious that they didn't need to. Usually, Molly stood back and so I would close the door. Clearly, Molly didn't need to relieve herself at that point in time. Immediately, Mary Belle would come into the room when she heard me letting some of the dogs outside and would attempt to force Molly to go with the others. "Molly!" she would shout at the cowering animal. "Molly, go on . . . go on outside! Did you hear me? I said *outside*! NOW!"

"Mary Belle," I'd say, in defense of the dog shaking with confusion, "if Molly had to go she would've gone out when I opened the door for the others. She doesn't need to."

"Oh yes, she does!" she'd bristle. "Go on, Molly!" And Mary Belle would begin to chase the dog about the house—sometimes actually getting hold of her collar and hitting her.

"Mary Belle, stop that!" I'd say, running to rescue the poor animal. "She doesn't have to go out. She's eight years old and knows when she has to go outside. If she didn't run out with the others she doesn't need to. Look how you're treating her. You're scaring her."

Mary Belle might stop at this point. She'd give me a crusty look, "You!" she'd spout. "You're just ruining everything!"

And poor Molly would hightail it up the stairs to hide beneath my bed, with Mary Belle sighing and getting angry over the whole incident. This might happen three times a day. I would actually catch myself trying to quietly sneak my own dogs outside, just to avoid an unnecessary confrontation.

The obsession with bladder function had also carried over to Mary Belle's own system. This seemed to appear in blocks of time. It would be an obsession for a couple of months and then seem to be forgotten for several more. It appeared to run in cycles for no reason. When it was in its active stage Mary Belle would wring her hands, sigh and moan, and complain that "she's having to run to the bathroom to urinate every five minutes all day long." When this new complaint first began, we had to admit that we hadn't noticed the frequency and Sally took her at her word. Sally took her mother to the doctor. He couldn't find anything wrong, but said that, if it continued, they'd run some tests.

After that announcement, Sally and I closely observed Mary Belle's "activity" during the day. We did this in a nonchalant manner, and it was not obvious to her that we were watching to monitor the frequency of her bathroom trips. She continued to bemoan the fact that she was tired of getting up and constantly going to the bathroom. We finally sat her down for a talk—for a reality check.

"Mother," Sally gently began. "Mary and I have been closely watching you for three days now. We've been especially concentrating our attention on watching how many times you've gone to the bathroom. We've been counting the trips you make during the day."

Mary Belle smiled. "See? Now you know that there's something wrong with me."

"No, Mom," she said, "you go to the bathroom less than either of us do. There's absolutely nothing wrong with you."

"Oh no," she adamantly insisted, "I have to go every five minutes. You two weren't watching closely enough. I'm so tired of it. Something's got to be wrong with me."

Though we tried and tried to tell her that we saw her go into the bathroom only three times throughout the entire day, she could not be convinced of that fact. All of our various attempts to help her see the reality of the situation were denied while she kept strongly insisting that "something was terribly wrong with her and maybe the *real* problem was that we just didn't care about her enough to find out what was wrong."

Sigh. Alzheimer's caregivers sigh a lot.

There was no way that Sally was going to put her mother through a battery of hospital tests for the problem of frequent urination when, in reality, it was so obvious that it was just not the case—that it was simply a matter of an Alzheimer's delusional obsession with bodily function. During the time that Sally and I gave special attention to this monitoring, we also noticed that Mary Belle didn't even physically carry out the behavioral "acting out" of her delusion by actually walking into the bathroom and sitting down on the toilet. She simply took the shortcut by *believing* she did this all day long. We'd observed her napping in her recliner for a couple of hours, wake up, and immediately begin bemoaning the fact that she "just finished going to the bathroom *again* and how weary it was making her." Yet she'd never left her chair.

Then, quite mysteriously, the bathroom obsession would leave as quickly as it had appeared, and we'd go for weeks without Mary Belle giving a single thought to having a frequent urination problem—she'd be just fine, just as she always had been during the obsession phase.

Sally was good at being attuned to her mother's physical condition at any given time. Just by looking at her mother, she could immediately tell if her blood pressure was high and she'd make her sit down so they could take a reading (the monitoring unit was never far away). When taken, it was usually way up there, and Sally would make her mother sit in her chair and relax for a few hours until the reading returned to a more acceptable range that allowed for low-level activities.

The frequent urination issue got us. It's not something you normally take special note of during your busy day, so, at first, we took her at her word but knew we needed to each keep one eye on her to monitor a full day's activity to determine the facts. In actuality, Mary Belle visited the bathroom far less than we ourselves did. Though we hadn't yet nailed down the spark that started up this specific type of obsessiveness, we did know that it was silently ticking away in her subconscious like some Twilight Zone clock that would chime the time for it to begin again as it moved through its cyclic gears.

Pacing. Pacing while Sally was away from the house was another compulsive activity. Nearly every ten minutes while her daughter was gone, Mary Belle would come over to the computer where I'm working and ask, "When will he be back?"

"Mary Belle," I'd remind her, "Sally's a woman. There are no he's in this cabin. Don't worry. She will come back home. I just can't tell you exactly when."

"Oh." And she'd return to her pacing pattern that encircles the stairway.

Five, ten minutes later she'd again be standing at my side, just silently standing there waiting for me to notice her.

It was hard not to notice someone standing beside me while I was sitting at a computer trying to write a book. I looked up at her face that reflected the urgent, hand-wringing question waiting to be voiced.

"Will he call if he's going to be late?"

I didn't bother going through the "gender" explanation again because it was futile. "She can't be late because she doesn't need to be home by any special time. She will come back home, Mary Belle. I just don't know when."

"Oh."

Pacing.

Circling. Circling.

At my side again. "Where did he go?"

"She didn't tell me. She had a lot of errands to do."

"Oh. When will he be back?"

And so went many of my days.

This behavioral example is the type that can cause the caregiver much frustration; yet, keeping in mind that the patient does not remember that she/he just asked the same question less than two minutes before is paramount.

Understanding. Understanding and having the acceptance of the conditions of the disease is a huge help that goes a long way towards maintaining that all-important patience with a capital *P*. Sure, it's frustrating for the caregiver to be constantly interrupted while trying to concentrate or work on something—especially if you're self-employed and have to devote a certain amount of that time each day to making your living. Sure it's irritating to be continually asked the same question over and over again, but your response to it will come easier and, eventually, it comes quite instinctually, once understanding and acceptance are gained. The patient is likened to a very small child.

As a caregiver, you learn to understand that actively demonstrating your frustration or outwardly displaying your irritation has no constructive effect on resolution or cessation of the offending behavior. No matter what your response is, the behavior will repeatedly occur, so you may as well make the situation less volatile and stressful by keeping a cool head. I will not go as far as saying we learned this the easy way. We all have our limits and can be pushed past them. But exploding and barking back at the patient only exacerbate the behavior, and you never want to initiate that through your own behavior. You learn that you can control many situations by way of your own responses. Gentle patience can often keep the behavior from getting out of control. It can prevent the patient's behavior from quickly turning into an anxiety attack or slipping into physical combativeness. Calm begets calm.

Though Mary Belle obsessed in many ways over a wide variety of subjects, the final example of obsessive/compulsiveness that she frequently exhibited seemed to be a nervous fascination with her rings. She'd sit in her recliner for hours, twisting the rings around her fingers and taking them off and putting them back on. Since Sally was a jeweler and goldsmith for many years and has a basement full of specialty tools, her mother would frequently go to her with a request.

"Will you make this ring smaller? Can you cut this ring off my finger? Where's my opal ring? Can you clean my diamond ring? Will you take this red (garnet) out of this ring and replace it with that green (emerald) stone?"

And Sally would usually stop what she was doing in order to comply with her mother's request—just to see a smile brighten up her mother's face.

The caregiver has to accept the multiple behaviors of obsessive/compulsiveness with grace. Those behaviors that may be physically harmful, such as picking one's nose, must be immediately addressed and can be gently diverted by shifting the patient's attention to safe behavior, such as using the tissue box. Those types of behavior that are physically harmless are accepted as being just that—harmless.

Paranoia and Phobias

Although it's known that many people in all walks of life can display behavioral traits that are associated with paranoia and phobia to some degree, the traits are common symptoms that have been shown to develop with the Alzheimer's patient. The individual who never had a suspicious bone in his/her body will suddenly exhibit outrageously paranoid thoughts and demonstrate related behavior when afflicted with the disease. Phobias set in and take hold as a rash of new fears rush to the fore of the patient's mind.

Simply defined, *paranoia* is the presence of unfounded suspiciousness and *phobias* are deep-seated fears. The variety of these two behavioral elements is great. The Alzheimer's patients may become fearful of being in a car, or may suddenly develop a fear of eating utensils, and, as a result, begin perceiving all foodstuffs as finger food. They might have a delusional fear that someone is going to come and take their pet or steal their identity. The range of these phobias seems to be unlimited.

So, too, are the targets of paranoia. The patients will exhibit an irrational and oftentimes passionate sense of suspiciousness regarding all manner of issues—suspiciousness associated with their money, with the credibility of all those they come in contact with, questioning the motives of others, and/or being leery of the medication they're handed.

Because of this behavior, there is a natural tendency for family and friends, and especially the daily caregiver, to feel as though their love and trust are being placed under deep suspicion. It's disheartening for them to see someone they love suddenly perceive them as being from the *Star Wars* Evil Empire. Yet, this is just another example of the disease's symptoms that must be seen through the eyes of rationality—of understanding and acceptance. Although the suspicions *appear* to be personally directed, when rationally viewed, one realizes that it's simply a "patient perception" that is broadcast over the breadth and length of his/her entire social spectrum. This becomes clear when closer examination of the behavior eventually proves that even the innocent mailperson, meter reader, and busy Federal Express delivery woman can be just as suspect as the caregiver or family member.

When the caregiver is exposed to this suspicion on a constant day-to-day and even hour-by-hour rate of experience, it can be difficult to maintain that all-important logical perspective, and the caregiver can easily find herself slipping into instances of expressed frustration and knee-jerk responses to the behavior. These are natural and shouldn't be one of those events generating instances of the "false guilt" that is known to frequently plague the Alzheimer's caregiver, family, or friends. Nobody said it was easy dealing with this type of escalating dementia, especially when you were never trained to be psychiatric nurses or attendants; and nobody said you had to be a saint to care for an Alzheimer's patient. So give yourself some slack when looking at your own responses to this type of behavior when it's directed toward you. It's not a matter of the patient getting personal with you . . . it's a matter of a disease.

Examples

I previously mentioned the example of Mary Belle having to listen in on every single telephone conversation we had in the house. As soon as the phone rang she'd immediately interpret the sound as a signal for her to get up from her chair and discover who the caller was. This was evidence of her paranoia (suspiciousness) based on the phobia (fear) that we were keeping calls from her. Also, she thought that we were always going to be talking about her to everyone. Therefore, she found it necessary to listen to everything said as a result of that false thinking. If Sally was talking to her brother, Mary Belle would stand beside her or follow her about the house to remain within earshot. In an effort to distract her and give Sally some privacy, I'd ask Mary Belle if she needed anything.

"No," she'd snap with a look of irritation that I'd taken her attention away from the business of listening to Sally, "I just want to be sure I get to talk to him."

"When Sally's finished, she'll give you the phone," I'd reassure her.

"I'm going to *make* sure," she replied.

This lack of telephone conversation privacy happened to be an issue with me, so I'd gently remind her what she was doing. "Mary Belle, it's really not polite to listen in on someone else's phone conversation. I know this place is small, but Sally deserves the same privacy you want for yourself. We don't listen in on your conversations when you're talking on the phone. You need to give us the same respect in return. Why don't you go into the living room and then she'll be sure to bring you the phone when she's through talking."

At this point Mary Belle might huff off into the other room as suggested or, more times than not, she gave me one of her glaring looks and defiantly stayed rooted right where she was. In the case of the latter, Sally would take this as a cue and walk down to the basement or out onto the deck with the phone and close the door behind her. That move only served to deepen Mary Belle's suspicion and she'd then scoff and pace about the house until she was eventually handed the receiver.

I've also touched on the issue of our Rolodex and calendar. Daily these were meticulously examined and carefully compared against her own. This behavior was generated from an unfounded fear of not having her own lists as complete as they "should" be. The trouble was that Mary Belle could no longer differentiate our listing of friends and family members from her own. Our personal friends, my daughters, and other family members got added to her own lists because she thought we, for some sinister reason, had purposely left them off her lists. Well, sure, we purposely left them off because those individuals were people she never had any need to call; she has no relationship with any of them. Yet her irrational thinking was that those *were* people she needed on her lists and, therefore, we were purposely keeping her lists incomplete.

Snooping. As any Alzheimer's caregiver will tell you, snooping is a common trait of the patient. Snooping is generated from the phobia of thinking you're hiding things from him/her and the paranoia that attends that fear. Mary Belle would take every available opportunity to go through our personal things, including desktops, drawers, purses, files, etc. She'd check through cabinets, sideboards, and china hutches; she'd examine the telephone notepad to see what was written down after each phone conversation we had, look over bank statements found on my desk, and make it imperative to scrutinize every piece of outgoing mail that was set out to take to town. If a piece of mail had Sally's return address label attached to it, Mary Belle would take the piece of mail from the stack and ask, "What is this of *mine* that you're mailing? I want to see what it is." One of us would have to grab it out of her hands before she began to rip it open. Again we'd have to explain that "Sally has the same last name as she does and that this is *Sally's* mail, not hers." That didn't ever prove very fruitful or satisfying as far as ending the issue. She'd give us that doubting look as much as to say that she didn't believe us, then would walk away shaking her head in disbelief. There's nothing you can do about it, short of opening up the sealed piece of mail to prove your point; yet that gets old after the first few times and, since the same suspicion will happen over and over again anyway, it becomes pointless to keep mutilating your outgoing mail by slitting the top open, showing her that the contents have nothing to do with her, and then having to tape it back up again. A better solution is to simply hide the mail somewhere until you're ready to go out the door with it. The trouble with that is that you frequently find yourself getting all the way into town before you remember that you had outgoing mail hidden in the house! The caregiver learns that some solutions create a lot more steps in the simplest of chores, but if those additional steps avoid possible combative confrontations, the caregiver goes the extra mile or two to take those steps.

When Sally returned from town with the mail, her mother would frequently follow on her heels in an effort to oversee the sorting of it. This came from a fear that she was not being given her mail, that we were keeping it from her. Well, we gave her what was appropriate for her to have. Learning from past experience, we came to the wisdom of "censoring" what we passed onto her. We used to give her everything that came with her name on it, until Mary Belle got combative over us refusing to mail back her many filled-out new VISA card applications and sweepstakes forms, that included her purchasing things she said she didn't want. Regarding the sweepstakes, we'd even sat down with her to read the small print aloud to her—the *"bulk* of the winning" amount wasn't due to be *paid* for thirty years! And did she think she really wanted to wait thirty years to receive it?

After we gave her one of the AARP newsletters, she became extremely agitated over some article about retirement funds and some new Social Security legislation. In reality, she couldn't manage to make heads or tails out of the articles and she mistakenly believed that she should be receiving monthly checks from the AARP organization. She'd gotten herself so worked up about this that she was firmly convinced that she'd been actually receiving those checks all along and that we were "taking" the funds. Sally and I spent an entire day trying to explain the article to her and that she did not receive any monthly checks from the AARP. She was convinced that she was *entitled* to those checks and we spent exasperating, repetitive hours and hours trying to make her understand otherwise. She was so riled about this issue that she tried to call the accounting firm she retired from to talk to an old friend about her "missing" checks from the AARP. But she couldn't manage to dial the number right. Finally, Sally dialed it for her. To Mary Belle's surprise, she learned from this old friend that she was *not* entitled to monthly checks from the AARP and that she was mistakenly believing so. Although disappointed to learn that we'd been right, she finally seemed satisfied enough to drop the issue.

So then, because of the Alzheimer's patient's growing inability to comprehend what is read, we found it necessary to censor the literature Mary Belle was exposed to. She received all personal mail and packages from family and friends. We gave her the magazines Tony subscribed to for her. She got all innocuous mail, but those pieces that might have had the potential to cause her confusion or extreme agitation, such as those that invited her to apply for a new VISA card, were set aside by leaving them out in the car to later retrieve and toss into the woodstove along with the rest of the paper waste we routinely burn.

Suspicion raised its untrusting head whenever medication was handed to Mary Belle. She'd accept the variety of pills in her hand and then make a big show of examining each of them before taking the glass of water we were standing there holding out for her.

"This one's new," she might declare with confidence. "What's that one for?"

"No, it's not new. You've been taking that for six months. It's the stool softener the doctor wants you to take. Remember?"

"No, I don't remember. It's new. What's it for?"

"It's the stool softener."

"Oh." And suddenly, out of the blue, she believes you. This is a prime example of the lightning speed that a suspicion can turn to belief, or vice versa. One minute the patient may be absolutely convinced that you're trying to slip her some ominous medication and, in the very next breath, will solidly trust whatever you're handing her. In the mornings when Mary Belle was handed her pills she might look at them and immediately ingest them, or she might take them and throw them across the room believing we were "trying to kill her." Whenever she did this last move, we had to scramble to locate every last tablet so one of the dogs didn't beat us to it. You never know which response you'll be presented with and, therefore, the caregiver soon learns to always, *always* expect the unexpected—that patient responses or perceptions will be inconsistent and continually remain in a state of flux. For the caregiver, unpredictability becomes normalcy.

Many of these symptoms will be seen to be crossover behavioral characteristics that blend into other symptomatic categories. The paranoid phobia regarding her believing that we were not feeding her dog was also a symptom of "delusion" (covered in an upcoming chapter). Many unfounded suspicions are generated from delusional thoughts so, naturally, throughout this book you'll find various interconnected behavioral elements that were discussed in several closely related chapters.

Money is a major issue for the Alzheimer's patient. In talking with friends who've also gone through the experience of being at-home caregivers for an Alzheimer's-afflicted loved one, money issues appeared to be a commonly recognized obsession with them. They may think people are stealing it from them. They may believe they have an unlimited amount in the bank (a loss of understanding quantity and value). And, like Mary Belle, they may believe that people (or organizations) should be sending them monthly checks that they're entitled to receive.

Every time I was at my desk reconciling our personal checking account against the statement, Mary Belle would stand a little ways away by the dining table (not more than four feet) and try to give attention to my bookkeeping activity. I understood that the clicking of the calculator keys was an attractive sound to her because she spent her life as a bookkeeper, yet I also understood that now she had additional interests in my activity. Instead of telling her to stop watching me, I would look up at her and ask if I could help her with something or if there was anything she needed. She would respond by shaking her head or saying that she was "just looking out the window."

Mary Belle believed that the checks that Sally and I jointly have were hers. This belief came from her state of confusion and waning rationality. Her *eyes* saw both names on the checks, yet her *mind* only picked out the "Mary" in my name and connected it with Sally's last name. By combining the unrelated parts of these two separate names out of context she came up with her own name. We went through an exasperating and exhausting day-long event after Mary Belle had taken all of our bills off my desk and hidden them, thinking we were using her name on all of our personal bills. We searched every nook and cranny of the cabin, looking for that stack of bills that I was about to write checks for. Because of that one incident, we learned to hide every one of our bills from her. And, consequently, Sally had to lock one drawer of her desk in which Mary Belle's separate accounts were kept safely together; otherwise, they'd be missing.

The fear of being placed in a nursing home was another grave concern Mary Belle had repeatedly displayed. Therefore, the suspicion that we were planning to do so was an ever-constant presence in her mind.

One day, shortly after we brought Mary Belle to live with us, Sally took her mother into Cripple Creek to treat her to a beauty shop adventure. She was going to get her hair cut and permed. The beauty shop is located in the back of an old, multi-storied brick building that, in the old nineteenth-century mining days, used to be a hospital. Today the building is a hotel called the Hospitality House with camping facilities on the grounds. When Sally pulled up to the entrance, her mother's eyes widened like saucers. "I'm *not* getting *out* of this car! You can't *make* me!"

Sally, having no idea why her mother was behaving in such a defiant and contrary manner, gently responded in a reassuring tone, "Mother, I'm taking you to get your hair done. We're here. I thought you were looking forward to doing that today."

With a blazing look that could kill, mother promptly replied, "You *lied* to me! This is *not* a beauty shop! I'm not getting out of this car!"

"Mother, the beauty shop's around back," Sally explained.

"You're lying! You're a *liar*, that's what you are!"

"Lying about what? What's this all about, Mother?"

"You must think I'm stupid or something. I *know* that this is a nursing home. You're going to get rid of me by putting me in here! Well . . . it won't work! It won't work because I'm not getting out of this car!"

"Mother. This is a hotel. In the old days it used to be the town's hospital. See the campers and RV vehicles parked all over? It's a hotel and campground now. The beauty shop's around in the back of the building."

"Likely story."

So Sally drove around back and pulled up in front of the beauty shop. "See the sign in the window?" she asked, while pointing to the building. "It says, 'Casino Cuts.' It's the beauty shop where I made your perm appointment."

They sat in the car for a time. After Mary Belle spent several minutes observing women of all ages coming out of the building with freshly coifed hair, she was less certain that her daughter was lying to her about the place being a nursing home. She then got out of the car on her own volition and acted as though she'd never doubted her daughter for a minute. "C'mon," she said, "I'm going to be late."

This one incident remained in Mary Belle's mind, and, forever after, whenever Sally frequently invited her mother to "ride along" on one of her errands or asked her if she "just wanted to get out of the house for a while and go for a scenic ride around in the mountains," Mary Belle was suspicious of the "real" reason—the hidden agenda—behind the invitation, thinking that, just possibly, this was *the* time her daughter was going to drop her off at some nursing home. This suspicion, generated from the fear of living in a nursing home, prevented Mary Belle from voluntarily going out and enjoying herself as much as she could have. And then she'd tell family and friends that, "I don't get out much. Sally never takes me anywhere."

We've also observed a fear of strangers coming to the house and, once, while we were working on a construction project outside the cabin, we found ourselves locked out. Mary Belle had turned all the deadbolts and we had to pound and pound to convince her to open the door—that it really was just us. Once convinced that we weren't strangers knocking at her door, she'd take a long time letting us in. Actually, unlocking the bolt frequently proved to be a difficult technical feat for her to manage.

I've previously mentioned the issue of hygiene difficulties we experienced with Mary Belle. Getting her to take a routine shower was an ongoing battle of the wills that sometimes led to physical combativeness. Some Alzheimer's experts will claim that this is a common symptom because the patient has developed a deathly fear of water. Whether it's a fear of water or just due to forgetfulness was unclear to us as patient observers because Mary Belle exhibited no noticeable aversion to washing her hands, getting a drink of water, or doing the dishes. From the behavior we observed, we tend to think she just forgot how long it had been since she had a shower, and then didn't believe us when we told her, so we had to resort to showing her the mark on the calendar to prove our point.

Cleanliness is not a priority for Alzheimer's patients, because they simply *forget* to wash their bodies, put on clean clothing each morning, brush their teeth, or clean their dental appliances. They forget when these important hygienic routine practices were done last and don't give a thought to the activities unless someone calls their attention to them. Because we'd seen such a dramatic increase in various irrational fears develop in Mary Belle, I didn't doubt that many patients do have a fear of water. We just had not seen this specific phobia in our patient.

It's extremely frustrating and emotionally hurtful for the caregiver, family, and the friends of the patient when they're made to feel they're not being trusted, that they're believed to be continually lying, or that all of their innocent actions are perceived as being subversive or reeking with some type of subterfuge or personal agenda. With Alzheimer's, the psychological elements of suspicion and fears are common associative facets, yet, when fully understood by those close to the patient, come to be accepted as part of the disease, just as paralysis can be associated with a spinal injury or blindness with diabetes.

Dealing with the related behavioral symptoms of Alzheimer's is getting accustomed to the idea of actually dealing with the symptomatic behavioral aspects of increasing dementia. The brain cells are deteriorating. Their numbers are declining at a rapid pace. The dementia will not get better, only worse (until a cure is found). And, consequently, symptoms can be expected to increase in severity as time passes. This is what family, friends, and the daily caregiver must ever keep in mind. It's nothing personal, it's never personal . . . it's just the disease. It's just how it is.

Complaining and Verbal Abusiveness

The onset of the dual behavioral characteristics of complaining and verbal abuse may not be initially recognized as associated with the disease of Alzheimer's by the family members and close friends of an afflicted loved one. The reason for this is that these traits may *precede* the usual signs of memory loss, which folks naturally tend to immediately connect with the disease, or, as is more often the case, these behaviors may simply become more noticeable than the increasing instances of forgetfulness that the individual is attempting to keep under wraps (and can be quite successful at it for an extended period of time). It's possible for someone to be capable of hiding his/her forgetfulness for a longer period of time than she is able to hold her tongue when impatience and irritation well from within. Controlling tempers and managing manners are basic elements of maintaining a generally accepted level of the performance of social graces and common politeness while interacting with others. These graces, and the individual's attention to them, quickly wane with the Alzheimer's patient. And the effects of this diminishing concern for expressed kindness and simple social respect can oftentimes be attributed by family members and friends to a newly developed "crotchetiness" in so-and-so's old age. Though many elders do indeed slip into a type of devil-may-care philosophy in their later years, a suddenly displayed attitude of "sharp-tongued" expressions may be generated from a more serious causal factor than merely becoming crotchety or finally throwing decorum to the wind.

Whether the behavioral characteristics of complaining and verbal abuse are an initial symptom that's noticed by family and friends, or whether it develops somewhere within another stage of the disease, every caregiver will be quick to identify it as a classic clinical trait. It would appear that, no matter what is done for the patient or how much one goes out of her/his way to accommodate them, or how much one strives to make their environment a pleasant one, there will always be something about the caregiver or the patient's living conditions to complain to others about. This behavioral tendency would seem to lead one to conclude that the patient is never satisfied; yet both Sally and I, as daily caregivers who have been continually exposed to this type of uncharacteristic behavior, tend to think more along the lines that the behavior is more of a bid—a psychological *need,* if you will—for attention and/or sympathy from others as the individual's focus on life centers more and more inward, on the self, as concern for others wanes at a rapid pace. This lessening concern for others, and for directing the basic expressions of politeness toward them, can be observed in a wide variety of new behaviors, such as tossing Christmas gifts on the floor, no longer wanting to send a family member a birthday present, beginning to call people names, and saying disparaging things about everyone they know.

The verbal abuse appears to have several psychological sources. After being the recipients of many of Mary Belle's seemingly spiteful barbs, we came to view them as her desperate way of holding on to the last measure of independence she had left—that of personal expression and opinion.

It's the one venue through which the patient perceives a means of having control of a situation or gaining the upper hand. These patients no longer realize that kindness holds greater power than mean-spiritedness. The pre-Alzheimer's patient may have never in her or his life uttered one unkind word, yet during the disease, become progressively spiteful and spew cruel statements to anyone who chances to be near them. And, oftentimes, these statements are generated from completely delusional thoughts, skewed perceptions, and imaginary events.

Examples

Some of the complaining behavior that we noticed with Mary Belle corresponded to the symptom that's associated with the loss of social graces that the Alzheimer's patients exhibit. When she received a Valentine's Day gift in the mail from her son, she was excited to unwrap it. After she opened it, she smirked, "What am I going to do with this? I don't want this!"

We were aghast at her rude and completely unexpected response, because, in truth, the gift was a darling stuffed Snoopy holding a heart-shaped box of chocolates. All of our cajoling couldn't change her mind. "Give it away," she ordered with finality. So, we put it in a plastic bag and stored it away. When Sally had to regrettably relay the incident to Tony, when he inquired how his mother liked his present, he naturally felt bad, yet he understood. He asked her if she would save it for him because his fiancée was into Snoopy, and she'd love to have it. So that's what we did. The next time Tony came to visit, he took the Snoopy back to North Carolina with him. With this particular aspect of the "complaining" symptom, there's no gratitude felt or expressed appreciation offered to others in response to being the recipient of their gifts or what is done for them. There will always be something to find fault with.

Oftentimes, the patients will make statements to indirectly convey their growing "grouchiness" through other means. Mary Belle filtered her opinions to us through audible communications with her dog. "Molly," she'd grumble under her breath, "we don't like it here, do we. We want to go live someplace else." Or maybe, while she was petting her dog, a sentiment would be expressed, such as, "Molly, they're mean, aren't they. They don't feed you. They let you starve."

Again, the caregiver has to give first consideration to the source and, it is hoped, has by now learned that the best possible response to hearing these indirect statements is to ignore them—pretend they were never said in the first place. By now the caregiver has developed a thick, leathery layer of skin over her/his emotional sensitivity in regard to these unkind comments; otherwise, the barbs have the potential to cause stinging injury if they're internalized as being personal instead of being a clinical aspect of a disease. It does no good to actively engage the patient in an attempt to correct the delusional statements, because this usually results in a confrontation that can, in turn, lead to increased patient agitation and physical combativeness.

A large part of the caregiver's work is to maintain emotional equilibrium, both for self and for the patient, and by turning a deaf ear to the mean-spirited comments that the patient makes, the caregiver can make the situation quickly dissipate like a morning mist, rather than turning it into a battle that will only end in frustration and add to the stress level of both parties.

Another example of complaining we'd experienced involved dog baths. Because our little Yorkies had long hair, they required more frequent bathing than Mary Belle's schnauzer did. I'd devote half a day to this chore. One by one, I'd put a Yorkie in the kitchen sink, bathe it, and then take it into the bathroom for drying and grooming. When I finished, Mary Belle would be dramatizing sighs of exasperation and giving me glaring looks. I didn't bother to address the behavior, because I anticipated it as soon as I set that first Yorkie into the sink. She thought that we were being mean, ignoring her dog if we didn't also give Molly a groom and bath whenever we cared for the smaller dogs. Yet Molly's care was very different. It was much more involved and took longer. She requires grooming shears to properly do her entire body, not just a brushing out like the Yorkies need. One of us had to get into the bathtub with Molly to bathe her. It's more of a chore and we didn't always have that kind of time every time we cared for the Yorkies.

So Mary Belle would put on this animated show. She would huff about the house and flash us those flaming, laser looks. Finally she wouldn't be able to contain her irritation any longer and she would complain, "You are just so *cruel!* I can't *believe* how *mean* you are! You ignore my poor Molly. She needs a bath, too."

And Sally would either explain to her mother that we'd been so busy that the Yorkies were way overdue for bathing, or that our dogs needed baths more often than Molly did, or that neither of us has the extra time to get to Molly right now.

Because of the growing inner focus on self that develops in the Alzheimer's patient, Mary Belle didn't care about our time. She gave no consideration to what we had to accomplish that day in respect to giving our attention to urgent errands or pressing business matters that had to be handled. She wanted her dog bathed and groomed *when she wanted it done.* Period. That was her only focus and she remained single-minded about it. So for days afterward, she would hold this deep grudge and refuse to speak to us. She once held onto it for so long that, two weeks later, we found her crying, actually sobbing. When we inquired as to the reason why she was crying, she responded with, "You're so mean to my dog. You ignore her. You won't give her a bath." That day we had a full schedule of business affairs to attend to, and, because of the time it took to do a proper grooming job on Molly, there was no way we could fit it in. Mary Belle sobbed and wrung her hands over the issue all day long.

Finally, Sally found a day when she could fit in Molly's care. She decided to surprise her mother and snuck the dog down into the basement, spent over an hour grooming her with the electric shears and then secreted her up into the bathroom for a good bathing. Sally came down the stairs with a big smile on her face. Molly, looking show dog perfect, scampered happily behind her. Sally went over to her mother. "Look, Mother! Molly's all groomed and clean! Isn't she pretty?"

Mary Belle gave one of her exasperated sighs and shook her head in total disgust. "You really take the cake! I didn't *tell* you to do that *today!*"

Sally's smile dropped like an acorn from an oak. "But you were upset the other day when we couldn't get to Molly—when the other dogs got baths, remember?"

"No, I don't! You're lying! Oh," she cried, crossing her hands over her chest, "oh, you've made me so *upset!* Who *said* you could give *my* dog a bath? What've you gone and *done* to her?"

Okay. Okay. So now's that golden time when you inhale that extra deep breath of calming air, quickly turn to the wisdom of silence while mentally throwing your hands up, and go about some other business at hand. *You walk away from it.* You ignore the new rantings that've begun about how "inconsiderate and bold you were to just go care for her dog without first asking for permission to do so."

No gratitude. Absolutely none. And, the wise caregiver soon comes to expect none in order to maintain a manageable stress level and a firm grip on her/his own sanity. Caring for an Alzheimer's patient, especially on a twenty-four-hour basis at home, is an ongoing exercise in unconditional goodness, acceptance, and perseverance. It's learning to keep your back well oiled, so that the incoming rain of irrational and delusional comments doesn't soak through to the soft heart and weigh down your precious sensitivities in drowning pools of futility.

As previously mentioned, the greater percentage of the patient's complaining is not expressed in a direct manner to the face of the individual in question, but rather behind his/her back such as to another person (or animal) who's present, or over the telephone to anyone who will listen. This is an example of the behavioral trait commonly known throughout society as "backstabbing." This term sounds like a very harsh one to use, yet, clinically, it's a valid behavioral characteristic commonly developed by the Alzheimer's patient. The term is precise; there is no other word to describe the behavior because the patient can be as sweet as plum pudding to your face, take a phone call one minute later, and begin telling someone how mean you are. We could also call this the "forked-tongue" syndrome. Some would call it "talking out both sides of one's mouth." No matter how one chooses to word the characteristic, it still comes down to a back-stabbing type of behavior which family, friends, and caregivers never quite get accustomed to experiencing. This is because, just when you think everything's been going fairly well and things have been reasonably sunny as far as the patient's care, comfort, and level of contentedness go, the patient's statements suddenly come at you like a lightning-fast right hook that lands square between the eyes, and your reaction is likened to hearing an earth-shaking clap of thunder bringing dark thunderheads and torrents of rain over your sunny-day perception.

We learned of this fact the hard way because we'd always given Mary Belle complete privacy when she was talking on the phone. Never overhearing what she was saying to people, we couldn't understand the outraged callbacks we began receiving from everyone she'd spoken to. From those indignant folks we heard anger over our not feeding Mary Belle. We got irate reprimands for letting her dog starve, verbal slaps on the hands for not taking her to church, for not getting her out enough, for making her do our dishes, and on and on. We were shocked into a speechless state of affairs after hearing all these people's accusations being flung at us. Where was all this ridiculous nonsense coming from? Mary Belle?

We needed to get to the bottom of this situation and nip it in the bud before it blossomed into some noxious, full-blown poisonous flower. We suspected the stories were coming from Mary Belle herself, so, instead of defeating our purpose by standing next to her every time she got on the telephone (causing her to alter what was said in our presence), we continued to provide her with the perception of phone privacy by installing an automatic phone recorder in the basement so we could discover what sort of nonsense she was telling people. Every time the phone rang and was picked up, the recorder began. We ended up with a lot of wasted tape filled with innocuous family and business conversations, but what we got from Mary Belle was the golden mother lode we were searching for.

When we listened to the playback tapes we were shocked. We were hurt. On the tapes, she'd lower her voice as in great secrecy and tell people only half-truths and wildly misleading statements.

These included, "He (Mary) won't let me drive my own car." But she didn't add that the *doctor* himself *ordered* her to hang up her car keys and *forbade* her to drive.

"He (Sally) doesn't feed me." But she omitted the part that she *refused to eat* her meals if she couldn't give half of them to Molly.

"I never get out anywhere." But she didn't tell the other person that she *refused* frequent *offers* to get out, because of her fear of being dropped off at a nursing home.

"He (Sally) doesn't give me any money." And then she didn't explain that she hid it, lost it, or put it in the trash basket or woodstove.

"They don't take me swimming anymore." And then she omitted the part about Mary Belle herself *refusing* to go swimming anymore because Sally wasn't getting into the pool with her (we couldn't afford a health club membership for both of them, yet we'd always be sitting poolside while Mary Belle was swimming).

"He (Sally) won't take me to church anymore." But she left out the part about her adamantly *refusing* to go to church anymore because she didn't like the priest, didn't like the fact that bearded, mountain men were drinking out of the same wine cup that she was supposed to sip from, that the building was too old and too chilly.

When finally confronted with the telling of these secretive, half-truths she told people, Mary Belle dramatically and adamantly denied ever saying them. She'd flatly deny making the statements and demand to know why *you're* being so mean to her by claiming that she'd said them. It became a circle dance that the caregiver learns not to step to, so we had no alternative but to take the time to speak with the patient's family and friends in an effort to explain the *other* halves of the statements that the patient conveniently left out, and also apprise these individuals of the common tendency of those with Alzheimer's to mislead others by speaking half-truths. Usually people will understand. Sometimes they don't. They don't because they're not living with it day in and day out and may think that you're only making an attempt to cover your mean treatment. Outsiders don't know—can't begin to imagine—the nonsense an Alzheimer's patient can verbalize with seeming sincerity and credibility. Just like the incident I previously mentioned when Mary Belle told Judy that we were building a "big addition" onto the cabin though, in fact, it was only a small, hand-built garden tool shed. Judy had taken the statement at face value, without giving any consideration to it perhaps being a gross exaggeration or a completely fabricated statement. This situation of half-truths and fabrications is common for the Alzheimer's caregiver to have to handle, and it has to be accepted as just being one element of dealing with the disease's daily maintenance.

Once, when we had taken Mary Belle with us to a social gathering, she loudly announced, "They didn't feed me breakfast!"

Without missing a beat, Sally immediately responded, "Well, Mother, why don't you tell all these nice people what I made for breakfast."

"What you made? What you made? Oh yes! You baked blueberry muffins. You cooked herb potatoes and big, stuffed omelets!"

No further comment on the subject was required. Everyone understood. We didn't bother to add that Mary Belle had carried her overflowing breakfast plate to the kitchen counter and refused to touch it for reasons that she refused to share with us at the time. The caregiver quickly learns when and how to draw the line to prevent a scene . . . especially in a public place.

Abusive language is not unexpected from the Alzheimer's patient, especially as the concern for the common courtesies and etiquette wanes in direct proportion to the escalating focus on the self. No matter how much you do, you'll be perceived as the Simon Legree of the household. Mary Belle would often instigate an argument over something. Perhaps it would be over insisting on going outside and standing on an icy porch in winter to watch her dog do its business. Well, part of the caregiver's job is to make sure that the patient doesn't do anything harmful to her/himself. Standing on an icy, wooden porch is not healthy, especially in one's nightgown when a full-blown blizzard is in progress.

Such incidents happened several times in our home. On one blustery midwinter evening, I discovered that Mary Belle had snuck outside and, feeling guilty for not having kept a closer eye on her, I rushed to the door to bring her back inside. I reached for her arms to guide her over the icy porch surface and she immediately scowled while yanking back her arm. "Leave me alone!"

"But Mary Belle," I tried to reason, "you can't be out here like that. It's freezing. It's snowing. And, it's dangerous to be on this ice. Come inside. Please." And I again reached for her arms to support her.

Again she pulled back. "Leave me be! I'm *older* than you. I know *best!* Don't *touch* me!" (Touching seems to be a big no-no for these patients and can be the trigger for a combative incident.)

I had no choice this time. For safety's sake, I did touch her. I firmly grasped her arms and had to physically guide her inside, while she fought hard to remain outside where she wanted to be.

Once back inside, I again tried to help her see the reality of the situation. "Mary Belle, you could've fallen out there and broken your hip or . . . your neck! You can't go out in weather like that."

With fire in her eyes, she spewed back in my face, "Don't *ever* tell me what I *can't* do! You are the *meanest* person I've ever met!" With that said, she strode into the living room, plopped herself down in her recliner, and fumed with steaming anger.

I let the incident roll off my back and returned to the book I'd been reading before it all began. Two minutes later, she got up out of her chair, pushed up her sleeve, and shot her arm beneath my nose. "Look what you've *done* to me. I have bruises! *You* gave me bruises!"

Sally had been in the office area on the computer, and, overhearing this accusation, came flying into the living room. "Mother! How dare you! That's not fair! That's being mean to go to Mary and say such a hurtful thing. She was just trying to keep you from breaking your neck outside! You have a lot of nerve blaming her for those bruises when it was *you* who stood out there in the snow like a child and *fought* with her. If you hadn't fought with her, *you* wouldn't have given *yourself* those bruises."

"I did no such thing."

End of confrontation. It's the end because the caregiver recognizes a futile situation when one occurs. Yet all evening Mary Belle continued to make an animated point of rubbing her arms and shooting me accusatory side glances.

Did I feel guilt over those bruises? Absolutely not, at least not a personalized type of guilt. I felt bad that her own combative behavior caused them. I felt sympathy towards this elder who could no longer distinguish dangerous situations from safe ones, that she voluntarily and frequently placed herself in circumstances that could cause her great harm. I felt disheartened that, sometimes, the gentle, physical guidance required for safety's sake often had to be turned into physical force generated by the patient's own refusal to be helped out of said dangerous situations. But I did not feel a "personal" type of guilt over the bruises that she had caused by her own combativeness in the face of her refusal to voluntarily extricate herself from a potentially harmful situation.

This same type of physically combative incident happened when we experienced another urgent situation. I had to forcefully pull her inside the house after she'd gone out as a mama black bear was ambling through the yard with her two cubs romping behind her. She was completely unaware of the danger she had placed herself in, and, therefore, strongly resisted me when she thought I was "telling her what to do." Even after I pointed the bears out to her, she was focused on not wanting to be *told* to come inside, rather than recognizing the danger of the bears.

The skin surface bruising couldn't be avoided when initial gentle guidance produced no results and we were left with no alternative than to tighten that grip to get her back inside out of harm's way, or lift her up off the floor when she had fallen. And then . . . then she would get on the telephone and tell people that "Mary (or Sally) put bruises on her arms"—but she would never explain why, she'd never explain that it was because she was fighting us and being combative over our efforts to insure her own safety, or her bruises came from one of us lifting her up off the floor after she'd fallen.

Bruises. Bruising. Elderly folks have thin, fragile skin. They bruise easily, very easily. When Mary Belle missed the toilet and fell down between it and the bathtub and Sally had to lift her up, Mary Belle's arms bruised terribly just from someone getting her into an upright position. When Sally had to pick her mother up out of the rocking chair that Mary Belle had been sitting in and had tipped it over onto the floor after falling asleep in it, she not only received bruised arms from being helped up, but also had a big knot on her head where she'd hit the closet door frame upon falling over in the chair. We had to keep Mary Belle in long-sleeved shirts because she'd received terrible arm and wrist bruises, even some broken veins that bled through the skin from the little Yorkies jumping up in her lap and landing on her hands and arms. Molly caused Mary Belle's skin to lacerate several times just by gently pawing at her arms and hands to get her owner's attention.

Verbal abuse. Anything and everything can come out of the patient's mouth. Anything and everything said needs to be taken in stride—with less than a grain of salt—by the caregiver (and family and friends, too). But for the caregiver, it's wise to refrain from donning an ego in the morning like she/he dons a set of clean clothing—that ego is best left on the bedside table where it's safe.

If you spent the day preparing a special four-course meal, it wouldn't be uncommon to hear the patient respond with, "You *expect* me to eat this *slop*?" (Mary Belle developed a habit of calling her meals "slop.") As though you've just set nothing more appetizing or filling than bread 'n' butter in front of her for dinner.

If you'd spent several hours cleaning her room she might come to you with some comment, "You are something else! You dummy, I didn't *tell* you to do that *now!*"

We might have been running errands for her all day, picking up her prescriptions and buying her activity projects (we're so far up in the mountains that we have to drive 80 miles round trip for this type of shopping), and, upon our return, she would immediately greet us with a scowl and get in our faces with, "You left me *alone* all day!" never bothering to take note of the respite caregiver we *paid* to sit with her while we were away. And then she would again, in a secretively whispered tone of voice, get on the telephone and tell someone that, "I'm left alone a lot. I'm left alone a lot to take care of all those dogs." Being "alone" to her meant that Sally and I were gone from the house. Mary Belle did not count the presence of the respite person who was there with her while we were away for a few hours.

Name calling becomes the norm. These names can be anything from "slut" to "slop" to "liar." When this first began we were quite taken aback, yet after it became commonplace, we got so that we didn't even hear it anymore. At first it pricked at our feelings; eventually we got to the point where it passed over us like a cloud shadow leaving no hurtful effects in its wake.

The caregiver must understand that he/she is interacting with someone who physically looks like an adult yet, mentally, is experiencing a retrograde level of intelligence and rationale, and is psychologically regressing to a stage of juvenile behavior. It's likened to caring for a three-year-old caught within an adult's body. Tantrums. Meanness. Physical combativeness. Pouting. Refusal to eat. Name calling. Childish behavior such as sticking out the tongue and making faces at people. Denial. Statements full of half-truths. Spitefulness. Attempted motions to strike your face. Lying. All of these and more are common behavioral elements associated with the Alzheimer's patient. All of these and more are everyday routine aspects of the caregiver's eight-hour day. For the twenty-four-hour *at-home* caregivers, they're a routine part of their *lives*.

Sundowning and Night Disturbances

One of the more specific clinical behavioral symptoms identified as being uniquely associated with Alzheimer's disease is what the professionals (researchers, physicians, and experienced caregivers) have termed *Sundowning*. Sundowning is, in turn, directly related to the phobic symptomatology of the disease in that it's directly connected to the *fear of approaching darkness*.

Visible signs of this phobia can begin to appear as early in the day as lunchtime because the patient knows that, by the time he/she eats the next meal of the day, the sun may be lowering. In most cases, the anxiety doesn't begin until around 4:00 P.M. and some patients don't begin to show signs of nervousness until supper time. Many times, the signals associated with the agitation of Sundowning don't arrive until just before dusk and intensify thereafter. Depending on the patient's individual personality, the signs can vary widely: Pacing. Wringing of the hands. Facial expressions displaying anxiety and worry. Raking the fingers through the hair. Restlessness. Repeated trips to the windows. Making a circuit of the residence to check and double-check the locks on the doors, etc.

This Sundowning would appear to precede a fear of the night or darkness and may be associated with the patients' additional clinical delusional element of the disease, whereby they may believe all manner of wild imaginings related to the dark night that encircles their home like an ominous shroud. Rather than perceiving the reality of that darkness as the naturally occurring cycle of a twenty-four-hour period, they view it as being "unnatural" and highly threatening. Therefore, their delusional imaginings, such as bad people lurking beneath the window ledges, monsters coming out of the darkness, someone "out there" wanting to break in and get them, and "murderers," are all strong ideological threads that are tightly woven into the phobic behavior. This last causal focus on murderers is a disease-specific one related to the fear of the night, because there is repeatedly documented evidence of Alzheimer's patients having a fixation on death, especially their own. Therefore, it's wise for the caregiver to anticipate the onset of these daily fears by turning on the interior house lights long before this activity would normally be necessary. This simple solution can greatly aid in warding off the patient's Sundowning anxieties (or at least serve to lessen their severity). We have exterior floodlights mounted on the sides and back of the cabin. These lights illumine the driveway, the entire back area of the near woods, and the dog yard. These, as it turned out, were a boon for lessening the night fears of our own afflicted loved one.

Night Disturbances. These are symptoms that hold hands with Sundowning. During the night the patient is frequently restless, afraid to sleep because of what or who might be "waiting out there," planning to gain entry into the house during that "time-of-greatest-opportunity" when an unsuspecting sleeper is most vulnerable to an intruder. These disturbances manifest themselves in a wide variety of ways. The patient might pace her/his bedroom floor all night; the individual may wish to have the television blaring for the sense of companionship it gives; if the patient has a pet, the individual may want to hold it all night or keep busy by attending to chores that involve pet care, such as taking it outside, feeding or brushing it (during the night hours). These behaviors are clearly telling efforts made by the patients to remain awake and be "ready for the unexpected," so no intruder can take them unawares. These behaviors indicate more than just a fear of intruder possibilities, they represent an actual *expectation* of the worst during the night hours. Sometimes the patients may exhibit such a deep-seated fear of the nighttime darkness that he/she is in actual denial of its existence and will get dressed in fresh morning clothing, while insisting that he/she must leave for work, as though it's time to get up and go about one's *daylight* activities.

This "work" is an imaginary job. To maintain an awake state during the night hours, the patients will have planned for this nightly eventuality by getting his/her sleep during the daylight hours. They usually won't actually get into their bed during the day, but rather doze for a couple of hours at a time in a chair.

Night disturbances, such as wanting to go to a job or perform other daylight activities, are especially difficult for the at-home caregivers, who need their sleep, but, instead, they're up and being forced to deal with the patient, who often becomes physically combative in his/her attempt to convince the caregiver that he/she "must get to work."

Examples

Mary Belle had the delusional idea that she worked in a shoe factory. She'd get up at 3 A.M., make her bed, get dressed for work, and, with purse in hand, leave her room. When she encountered the locked gate at the top of the stairway, she'd forcefully push and pull on the door. When that proved futile, she would begin kicking it. She'd kicked it so forcefully that the metal plate of the latch bent. Of course this commotion instantly woke up the entire household.

Dogs were making a racket barking at the noises and we were forced to get up and deal with the situation. Words of reason weren't an effective solution when the event was that far gone, because attempting a calm resolution would sound something like the following scenario.

"Mother," Sally would sleepily say, "what are you doing?"

"I'm going to work! Those people are picking me up. They're waiting out there for me."

"No mother, you don't have a job. You're retired, remember? Nobody's out there waiting to take you to any job."

Then Mary Belle would become sarcastic. "You dummy, you slob, a lot *you* know. Now open this door!"

Sigh. "Mother, it's three in the morning. All the shoe factories are closed now."

Suddenly the gate would be given another hard kick.

"Mother! You're tearing my house apart. Stop it! Stop trying to break things!"

"Well, smarty slut, you won't let me out to go to work! What am I supposed to do?"

Right about at this point I would have heard enough and come out of the bedroom to see if I could be of assistance.

"Mary Belle, c'mon," I sighed, while reaching for her arm to guide her away from the gate, "let's get back to bed."

She yanked her arm back so hard and quick that she ended up hitting her hand on the wall. Daggers flew from her eyes into mine. "Now look what you've done, you slut! You hurt my hand! You leave me *alone!* Slut, that's what you are, nothing but a slob, slut." (For some reason, she came to love using that word.) "I need to go home!"

"What about work?" I asked.

"I have to go to work first. He's out there waiting for me. Then I'm going home."

Sally gently, but firmly, took one of her mother's arms while I took the other and we led her back into her bedroom. We entered the room with her and closed the door behind us, refusing to leave until she got herself back into bed. This might take a couple of hours before Sally's mother got tired of having us hang around in her room and resign herself, just to get rid of us. Mary Belle would begin crying while undressing and getting her nightie back on, all the while making sure we heard about what terribly horrid people we were for keeping her from her job and how badly she wanted to go back home.

"This is your home," Sally reminded her.

"It is?" came the surprised response.

"Yes, Mother, you've been living here for over three years."

"I have?"

I smiled at her and tried to sound chipper in an effort to raise the overall mood of the situation. "Sure you have, Mary Belle." I chuckled. "Remember when you wore your cowgirl hat and rode out here in the big moving van with Molly on your lap? Remember all the snow that was here when you finally arrived?"

"Nooo. No, I don't recall that." She paused for a few heartbeats to think about what I'd said. Then, "Well!" came the reply, full of a lightning switch to an attitude that was dripping with sarcastic indignation, "nobody ever *bothered* to tell me that! Guess I don't *count,* because that's the first I've heard of *that* one! Are you sure?"

"Yes, Mom, we're sure," Sally added.

"Well," Mary Belle sighed, while pulling the bed covers over herself, "I really don't know why I'm living off you nice ladies. We're not even related. I should be living with someone I'm related to. I should be living with family."

Hearing that, my heart ached for Sally. I could only imagine how a daughter must feel to hear that type of comment coming from her own mother.

Sally immediately responded with reassurance. "Mother, we are related. I'm your daughter. You live with me. This is my house. I own it with my friend, Mary. You live with us. You *do* live with family."

This news brought a smile to Mary Belle's face. Then she took the time to study each of our faces as though she was seeing us for the first time. The smile downturned into a frown. "Oh. Well then," she asked, "why aren't you in bed then? Go on. Get out of my room and go to bed so I can get some sleep! This is *my* room. You're keeping me up."

Incident over.

The incident was over, yet our entire sleep cycle had been disrupted and the event might have taken several hours to come to a satisfactory conclusion. It may be seven or eight o'clock in the morning by the time she wants to go back to sleep and, by then, it's time for you to get up for the day because a business call is already ringing on the downstairs phone.

The dogs are anxious to go outside and they're whining to get your attention. You let them out and go about brewing the morning's pot of coffee.

Your patient is upstairs happily snoring and you're bleary-eyed from lack of sleep.

You place a return call to the party you didn't quite connect with before the phone stopped ringing and try very hard to sound awake and rational.

When Mary Belle finally rises for the day, she will not remember the incident, and, with deep suspicion, will look at you as though you're fabricating the whole thing if you tell her about it. She may call you a "damn liar." It may be true forgetfulness or it may be denial.

Denial. It happens a lot. You don't bother trying to convince her of the incident because you've got a full day ahead of you and she wouldn't believe you anyway.

This behavior of not recalling the night disturbances was so frustrating for us that Sally actually entertained the idea of videotaping the events to prove to her mother that they did indeed happen. But what caregiver wants to add the work of taping an event when they have to be involved with dealing with the situation while still half asleep? That idea got nixed real fast, especially when we realized that we didn't even own a video recorder. We weren't about to go purchase one just for that purpose.

Another form of night disturbance incident would be when Mary Belle wanted the household to be up and active for the day at 2 A.M. She'd be dressed and standing outside in the hallway whistling. The whistling accompanied, "Doggie! Here, doggie, doggie!" She knew that our dogs were sleeping in the bedroom with me and she tried to get them awake and barking in order to get me up. This was not appreciated. This was definitely not appreciated because, many nights, I'm up late writing and may have just gone to bed shortly before she begins her whistling outside my door. So again we had to convince her that 2 A.M. was not the time to be getting up for the day. This convincing might take several hours.

Wandering during the night is another form of night disturbance that the Alzheimer's patient will commonly exhibit. Before we installed the gate at the top of the stairs, we'd find Mary Belle outside heading toward the moonlit woods or sitting in one of the vehicles having a conversation with an imaginary man. More on this in the Wandering chapter.

The final type of night disturbance we experienced with Mary Belle was screaming in her sleep. I have to admit that the first time this awoke me in the middle of the night, it was quite unnerving because she emitted a sound quite unlike human screaming. Mary Belle would make a sound like some wild animal howling and it would send chills through us. She often flailed her arms while howling, and knocked things off her night table and put bruises on herself after striking the headboard or her table. This behavior could happen as often as several times in one night or as seldom as once a week. Sally would race to her mother's side and wake her. "Mother, you're having another nightmare. What were you dreaming about?"

"Men" would always be the reply. Some man or men were after her and she was beating them off. And after Sally calmed her mother by showing her that she was perfectly safe in her own bed, Mary Belle would quickly fall back to sleep . . . only to have it happen an hour later. Leaving the bedroom lights on didn't appear to prevent those incidents from recurring.

The Sundowning syndrome is not an Alzheimer's symptom that is ever completely resolved, but it can be dealt with through management techniques that may ease patient anxiety and stress levels. When the sunrays begin to lengthen, the caregiver can take the patient outside and exclaim over the beauty of the late afternoon sunshine; perhaps a particularly beautiful sunset is beginning to display itself. Turning fear into an attitude of appreciation can go a long way to alleviate the anxiety the patient is beginning to feel at this specific, critical time of day. Sitting outside on porch chairs or going for a short walk can lift some of the phobia. Oftentimes, facing those fears will ease the anxiety. We're fortunate enough to have mountain wildlife come around after dark. Our floodlights illumine their presence. At night we took Mary Belle over to the window and showed her the raccoons lounging in the sunflower feeders or sitting on the porch eating from the scrap bowl we keep full for them. We'd take her to another window and point out the cluster of mule deer eating the sweet feed by the birdbath in the side yard. We drew her attention to the buck's antlers by smiling and marveling over their large size and many points. If she had something of high interest—of an innocuous nature—to look out at, she'd exclaim with delight over seeing such sights, and gazing out into the night became less fearful for her.

The caregivers, family members, and friends must be creative in the management of their patient or parent. There are alternative responses one can make to help that patient or parent experience less anxiety and stress when such symptoms as Sundowning appear. Understanding and creativeness can go a long way in making life easier for all concerned.

149

Demanding and Belligerence

It is not unusual for Alzheimer's patients to display negative forms of behavior that others would normally associate with an especially self-absorbed supreme monarch. Again, this may sound harsh, but the intent of this book is to deal with the common clinical behavioral characteristics of someone afflicted with this disease, and the growing focus on oneself is an identified element of Alzheimer's.

This strong psychological central focus on the self redefines the self-perceived character of the patient's image—that of the "Queen Bee" or the "Royal King" of the household, who makes enough demands that those closely associated with the patient may begin to feel as though they've been relegated to the position of personal subservience. With this disease, this is a recognized patient trait and attending caregiver/family responsive reaction.

The demands increase in accordance with the lessening level of patient recognition for other people's personal life responsibilities, individuality, or rights. And the patient's belligerence quotient rises as he/she is faced with opposition to being constantly waited on or entertained. This behavioral symptom works in direct tandem with the possessiveness element of the disease. The patient's ego becomes a growing force which the entire world is perceived as having to revolve around: not only is everything theirs, but every *person* exists for their whims. It's a little like the reverse of autism—instead of shielding the ego and internalizing the world by wrapping it around the self, the Alzheimer's patient will behave in the opposing manner by broadcasting the ego and externalizing it out into the world—like casting a personal ego net over all they see.

Evidence of this demanding symptom comes in many forms, shapes, and sizes. Naturally, it will touch on several of the other symptoms such as verbal abuse, combativeness, and first response denial. Yet the most identifiable associative behavior is belligerence. When the patient does not receive an immediate "expected" response to a demand (one that satisfies), he/she may become belligerent and difficult to manage. Using reason rarely reverses the situation and, through experience, the caregivers discover that the best response is to flat out state that they're there to *help* the patient, not to *wait* on their every whim. Some ground rules need to be established at the outset. By using this logic, the caregiver's ploy usually halts the behavior cold. The patient will act indignant and perhaps pout for a while, but further confrontation is avoided, and the situation is kept from being exacerbated by futile verbal discourse over the incident.

Belligerence can raise its head many times throughout the day. One reason for this is because Alzheimer's patients don't like to be told what to do. They especially detest being told what they *cannot* do. This is why the caregiver quickly learns how best to phrase communication. If the caregiver says something like, "You can't use knives anymore," the patient's ire will rise and he/she will belligerently reach for that knife out of spite. So, instead, the caregiver words it differently so as to maintain a calm and unriled patient, "I just sharpened that knife. Here, let me do that for you. I wouldn't want you to cut yourself." The patient, hearing that type of response, shifts the reaction from one of belligerence to one of satisfaction, "Oh, how nice that you care about me and want to wait on me!" The caregiver's response is important. If the caregiver had said, "You can't use knives anymore, or you're not *allowed* to use knives anymore," then the patient would most likely have become indignant and reached for the knife and, quite possibly, become aggressive with it and used it to threaten the caregiver. There could've been a physically combative incident over it, resulting in someone getting injured.

The Alzheimer's patients' families and friends, especially the daily caregivers, have to be pseudo-psychologists who are constantly on their mental toes, maintaining a finger on the pulse of the patient's continually altering frame of mind. By keeping this psychological awareness honed to a razor-sharp edge, the caregiver avoids many unnecessary confrontational incidents and bolsters a more even keel (and manageable) attitude with the patient. By doing this, the relationship between the two individuals experiences less dips along the road they're traveling together.

Examples

One autumn evening around eight o'clock when Sally and I were sitting in the living room, vegging out after spending a long day cutting down diseased trees in the woods, splitting, and stacking them, Mary Belle appeared in front of Sally with her jacket on.

Sally looked up at her mother and asked, "Are you cold?"

Mary Belle replied, "No, I'm not cold. I'm waiting for you to take me gambling!"

"Gambling! We're not going down to Cripple Creek. Where'd you get that idea?"

"Well, I *want* to go! You're taking me gambling *now!*"

With exhaustion heavy in her voice, Sally sighed. "Mother, look at us," she said, pointing over to me, "we've been cutting wood all day long. We're tired and we're full of sawdust and dirt. We're just resting until we can go take showers. There's no way we're going out anywhere tonight."

"I want to go," she said, turning to cross the room and sit in her recliner. "I'll just wait for you two to put your coats on."

I glanced over at Mary Belle. "You're going to have a long wait. You might want to take your coat off so you don't get hot."

"I'm fine," she sarcastically shot back. "You won't be that long."

After half an hour of looking back and forth between Sally and me while emitting great dramatic sighs, she crossed the room again to stand before her daughter. "You ruined everything! You *always* ruin *everything* for me!" And she kept her coat on until bedtime.

This singular incident clearly exemplified the Alzheimer's patient's lack of consideration for those around them. Mary Belle gave no thought to how physically tired we were. She got it into her head that she wanted to go to a casino, and that's what we were going to do, come hell or high water. As an aside, when Mary Belle first came to live with us and her disease wasn't as far advanced, she loved going gambling. She absolutely loved it. She'd previously been to Las Vegas and was well acquainted with the various gaming activities the casinos offered; and, in Kansas City, there were casino boats on the river.

During her early months with us, she loved playing video poker and was good at it. She preferred playing the quarter and dollar machines and wanted us to take her several evenings a week. She perceived it as not just a fun activity and a possible opportunity to come home with more money in her pocket; she also greatly enjoyed the glitzy atmosphere, the lively music, and the social contact when we ran into people we knew there. At that time Mary Belle was also adamant about people not knowing how much she was spending at the casinos, or about the large monetary gifts she'd given to people; whenever friends or family asked her if she'd been down in Cripple Creek "playing," she'd immediately deny going and respond with, "Oh no, no, I don't go down there." Yet on a weekly basis—sometimes several times a week—she'd tell Sally to go get her more money and Sally would just write a check at the casino and hand over the cash to Mary Belle to spend. She'd tell us not to say anything to anyone because, according to her, "My money and what I want to do with it is nobody's business." Later, it was different.

Later, when we took her to a casino after she expressed an interest in the activity, she was not capable of playing her favorite video poker anymore and we would find her a simple nickel slot machine to sit at. She immediately forgot what button to press. She would be bored after five minutes and walk away from her machine, leaving as much as 1000 credits in it. She would wander around the casino, dropping her dollar bills, and leaving a paper trail of money on the floor behind her, or leave her purse somewhere and then want to go home within twenty or thirty minutes of arriving. Taking her to the casinos became an activity we avoided unless it was to take her out for a nice dinner; then we'd walk directly to one of their restaurants.

This one example specifically depicts the common Alzheimer's patient's behavior of demanding to be taken somewhere and then, when taken, wanting to turn right around and return home. Likewise, when outings are offered by the caregiver, the patient will refuse them and, afterward, tell people that she's "never taken anywhere." However you cut it, it's a Catch-22 situation for the caregiver.

Mary Belle expected "first deference" given to her in all situations. If you set a dinner plate down in front of someone else before she'd been given hers, you'd receive a glaring look, or perhaps she'd get up and flatly refuse to eat at all. If she did decide to eat, she would dramatically inspect each edible item on the plate—each pea, each kernel of corn—as though looking for imperfection or something suspicious hidden within the mashed potatoes or spinach. If we made an extra special dinner by placing fresh-cut wildflowers on the table, lighting candles, and using placemats beneath the plates, she'd refuse to come and eat when called to dinner because we hadn't *delivered* her plate to her lap in front of the television. Then she'd say that we "ruined dinner by putting it on the table."

Another way she thought we "ruined dinner" was if Sally and I were involved in construction projects and were too busy to take the time out to formally eat, or if we were just not particularly hungry for lunch or dinner, and one of us would fix just Mary Belle something. She'd be outraged that no one was "dining with her" and, consequently, would refuse the food we took the time out to fix.

Though we almost daily reinforced the fact that it was Mary Belle's home just as much as it was ours, and that any food in the refrigerator and cupboards was there for her to freely take from whenever she felt so inclined, she flatly refused to help herself. Instead, she would come to one of us and ask, "Are you going to feed me or not?" We would again tell her that she was always welcome to take whatever she fancied from the kitchen. She'd sigh and walk away without getting herself anything. Sometimes we'd let that go without stopping what we were doing to fix her something because, at every opportunity, we were trying very hard to help her maintain some sense of self-sufficiency and give her something to do.

She often complained of having nothing to do, but when we suggested she get herself something to eat, she refused. She refused with, "*You're* supposed to fix it *for* me!" If we attempted to explain that we were trying to give her an activity to do, or that we wanted her to keep up her living skills, she would give us that "incredulous" look as if she believed we were lying to her. She would not get herself as much as a donut from a package or an apple, grape, or banana from the fruit bowl sitting out on the counter (even when we frequently reminded her of the importance of eating bananas for the potassium they contained).

Belligerence goes hand in hand with the "demanding" trait of Alzheimer's. When one makes demands and those demands are not immediately satisfied, the belligerent behavior follows as a natural course of response to the inaction that was not expected. The belligerent behavior is likened to the response of a small child who doesn't get what she wants.

Belligerence with Alzheimer's means: "I want what I want when I want it and . . . I'd better get it or else!" The caregiver understands this juvenile attitude in the patient and, through trial and error, discovers ways to sometimes circumvent it, which doesn't always work because of the iron-like tenacity of the patient who holds onto his/her idea with a white-knuckled grip. The "I will get *what* I want *when* I want it" idea appears to be a common attitude related to the disease's behavioral characteristics and, because of it, can quickly lead to verbal abusiveness and/or physical combativeness by the unsatisfied patient.

I've seen Mary Belle become so frustrated over Sally or myself not jumping the second she said, "jump!" that she would raise her hand to slap our faces. She made the beginning motion—a few months after that, she actually began following it through to hit her mark.

In belligerence she'd throw a full plate of dinner down on the floor after being gently reminded that the food was for *her* nourishment, not her dog's.

When cautioned not to go outside because the black bear had been in the yard several times that morning, she'd bristle and keep going to the back door to open it and go out.

She detested that she was no longer allowed to drive, so she kept trying to quietly sneak out of the cabin and get behind the wheel of one of our vehicles (we learned to remove the keys we'd always left hanging in the ignitions).

There were times when Mary Belle would become so belligerent over something that she'd just walk out the cabin and up the drive. (Remember, though, this drive winds a quarter-mile through deep woods.) A walk up our drive is not like most people's. Not only was it strenuous for her heart, the driveway contained a vast array of potentially dangerous wildlife. Mary Belle suddenly could have found herself caught between a mother black bear and her cubs.

Belligerence was when she would sit with her coat on all evening after we didn't take her where she suddenly announced she wanted to go. It was holding a grudge all day long for not letting her go to her imaginary shoe factory job at 2 A.M. It was refusing to eat all day because you didn't fix her breakfast eggs just right. It was all these and countless more behavioral events that exemplify just how childishly an Alzheimer's patient can respond to not getting her/his way.

For the caregiver, this childishness is best managed by being overlooked. When Mary Belle defiantly sat all evening with her coat on while waiting for us to take her somewhere, we completely ignored the fact that she was wearing it. Oftentimes belligerence, such as the wearing of the coat, was enacted for the purpose of getting a rise out of others. When that rise doesn't happen, the patient's balloon develops a slow leak and, eventually, it amounts to nothing more than a leftover residual effect that has lost its former punch. Again, it's the caregiver's responsive reaction to belligerence that can inflate or deflate a potentially explosive situation.

Shadowing

Shadowing is a term the Alzheimer's experts have classified as a recognizable disease behavioral symptom. Shadowing means "following." These patients have a common tendency to follow others around. For the at-home caregiver, this can be a frustrating and irritating behavior which adds to their diminishing opportunities for personal privacy.

This desire to follow others may come from one of the many Alzheimer's-related phobias (a fear of being left alone, for example). It may be generated from a paranoia, a suspiciousness that needs constant verification by continually "watching" another person to "catch them in the act" and prove out their delusional suspicion. It may be caused by a newly developed psychological need to know what everybody around them is doing. Whatever the reason for the behavior, it must be accepted by others as a condition of the disease and not taken personally.

Examples

I've previously mentioned the fact that Mary Belle would frequently stare at us. Whether we were trying to relax in the evening with a good book, or involve ourselves in a good movie on television, she'd fix her sights on us and hold them like a magnet. Sally and I have always had the same habit of getting our morning's cup of coffee and sitting in the living room, surrounded by our own personal, quiet space and just "vegging" in it until we're awake enough to have conversation or begin our day. Mary Belle would stare at each of us in turn while we were trying to stay in our little "wake-up" spaces. It was terribly unnerving and certainly detracted from any sliver of leisure or privacy we were trying to achieve.

Frequently, when I was working on a book manuscript at the computer, Mary Belle would come and stand behind me for half an hour, or she might have decided to sit down at the dinner table just a few feet away from the office area (the cabin is small) and stare directly at me while I was desperately trying to get just the right wording for a philosophical thought. At first, her staring at me was not conducive to maintaining my focused train of thought or to composing text with ease. But through the necessity of dealing with the reality of that daily behavior, exercises in concentration paid off. I could completely disassociate the activity of utilizing the mental thoughts involved in writing on the computer from the mental distraction of Mary Belle's constant stare while I was working. However, I was unable to completely relax while she stared at me during my attempts to achieve some evening leisure time with a good book. This inability was certainly not from a lack of trying. I tried all the personal types of amenities that usually serve to sooth me: burning cedar or patchouli incense, lighting candles, having the lights down low, and even listening to soft music with headphones on while reading, but still she stared—still I was aware of that constant stare and distracted by it. So if it was summertime, I would take my book out onto the deck; if it was winter, I'd retreat to my bedroom or to the basement lounge chair with the book.

Staring at you while you were on the phone was resolved by taking the phone with you into the basement or up to the bedroom.

Her habit of staring at people in public, such as in restaurants, was more difficult to control because you had to openly address the offending behavior. You had to softly remind her that she was being rude, that she was not using polite manners in public, and that her staring was making the other diners uncomfortable. At this point, because she was being told that she "couldn't do something," she might have denied that she was doing it, even *while* she was doing it.

Staring at others is an associative element of the Shadowing syndrome connected to Alzheimer's disease. Staring is a "connective" venue for the patient. It connects the patient to another individual and, therefore, proves to be a psychological aid that helps them to feel less alone and isolated.

Shadowing is the act of physically following another individual around. Mary Belle's performance of this specific behavior appeared to fluctuate according to each day's particular sense of psychological need. Some days she'd only follow us with her eyes or ears, other times she'd actually be physically hard on our heels all day. More than once she was so close behind me that I nearly toppled over her when I turned around.

If Sally and I were in the basement workshop, involved in the metal sculpture work that we began as a side business for extra income, Mary Belle would continually open the stairway door and attempt to descend the stairs. We had to remind her that the basement was off limits to her because the stairway has no handrail and she risked falling every time she tried to come down. So we countered this negative reason with a positive suggestion and followed it up with something like this, "We need you to listen for the phone," or "Will you watch the dogs for us while we're working down here?" This gave her purpose. It gave her a reason to stay upstairs and have something meaningful and constructive to do—feeling helpful—and, unless she was in a particularly belligerent frame of mind, that would be enough to satisfy her and solve the problem.

It doesn't take a nuclear physicist to understand that being followed around all day—or for most of the day—greatly robs one of any sense of personal privacy. Your home is your sanctuary, or at least it's supposed to be. Your home is the one place where you're normally assured the simple right of enjoying complete privacy, yet by having an Alzheimer's patient in that home, that sanctuary is entirely eliminated and you're forced to grow accustomed to the fact that you constantly have eyes on you, or that someone is standing directly behind you at all times, or that all of your conversations are being overheard.

Think about that. Think about being at home and continually having a set of eyes on you. Perhaps my use of the word "accustomed" is a bit optimistic, for you never truly get used to the idea, you never really become comfortable with the situation, but you're always aware of it just the same.

My attempts at respite out on the deck during sunny, summer days were, more often than not, shattered when Mary Belle would follow me out there and then let all the dogs join her. The peacefulness of the forest surrounding the cabin was sharply rent by the dogs' playful barking at the squirrels and romping about in play. If I went back inside, the whole gaggle would follow on my heels as one shadow. So you stay where you are, let out an accepting sigh, and laugh at the pups' amusing antics. If you don't internally work with the situation by having *acceptance* for reality, all the bucking in the world will not bring you one iota of the peace you're initially seeking.

In the above example I gained the joy of watching our little furry people romp and play. I merely accepted the necessity of exchanging one form of relaxation for another. In the end, I achieved the same purpose—that of enjoyment. Laughter instead of solitude.

The one instance in which Sally had a particularly difficult time dealing with her mother's penchant to shadow was when she was involved in busily preparing a meal. Sally loves to cook. It's a given that it's her kitchen. It's also a given that good cooks don't like to be bothered or have someone underfoot every time they turn around during meal preparation. Each time Sally began to prepare a meal, Mary Belle would be right there watching every move over her daughter's shoulder. Not only was every move watched, every move was questioned. Sally's never been long on patience, yet I give her a lot of credit for expending the energy to push it beyond her normal limits when it came to her mother. She went the extra mile.

"What's that?" Mary Belle asked of a spice she saw taken from the cupboard.

"Dill seed."

"What's it for?"

"Flavoring."

"Why?"

"To make the meal taste better."

"What's that?" her mother asked again, noticing another spice being used. "Now what're you doing?"

Sally bumped into Mary Belle as she turned to add the new ingredient to the skillet. "Mother, will you please give me some room to move around?"

Not moving, "Aren't you going to add celery seed, too?"

"No."

"Why not?"

"Because celery seed doesn't go into this."

"Does so."

Sally turned to reach for the ladle and accidentally stepped on Mary Belle's toe.

"Ouch!" Mary Belle bitterly exclaimed, looking down at her foot. "You hurt me!"

Sigh. "Mother, I can't prepare this meal if I'm always bumping into you. If you have to watch, please stand back a ways so we're not stepping on each other's *toes*."

And, Mary Belle, with lips firmly pursed in an exaggerated pout while dramatically hobbling away, would move back a few paces to stand in front of the refrigerator. This was okay until Sally needed to retrieve the sour cream from it.

Mary Belle moved again . . . right in front of the steaming pots *on the stove.*

So then. What's the solution to this type of problem?

A distraction. Find something of interest for her, maybe on television. I'd be aware of the growing problem transpiring in the kitchen and call Mary Belle into the living room to come see the pregnant squirrel at the feeder or some type of new bird species. Usually the distraction would be enough to hold her attention and she'd completely forget about returning to her self-appointed job as cook supervisor. Yet when she wanted to follow one of us into the bathroom, that was going a yard too far, and we had to firmly remind her again about politeness and respecting another individual's right to basic privacies.

Shadowing makes other people, especially the caregiver, feel as though they've suddenly developed a human extension attached to them. Whether that extension is in the form of a physical body on their heels or in the form of eyes staring at them, it's something one must accept and adjust to in order to effectively manage and deal with the behavior. It's a behavior that isn't going to go away any time soon; if anything, it's only going to get worse. Realizing that fact makes the caregiver a mistress of creativity.

When Sally and I were outside working on cabin projects and Mary Belle was right there wanting to help, we came up with simple activities she could do without compromising her physical health. For example, when we were hammering in loose nails on the cedar siding, we'd purposely drop some and ask her if she could help us out by checking the ground for any stray nails that might have fallen. When Sally was cutting wood and I was stacking it, I'd hand Mary Belle the kindling-sized pieces and she'd be as happy as a lark setting them on the growing pile of cordwood.

Mary Belle liked to be doing whatever we were doing. That's normal. It's a normal form of companionship and camaraderie.

She loved having that sense of "joining in." The quintessential example of this was when Sally and I actively took on the massive job of staining the entire cabin last summer. We'd repeatedly tried contacting various construction men to come give us an estimate for the job, but kept getting put off with one excuse after the other. Finally, we decided to save big bucks by doing the job ourselves. The weeks of summer were slipping away and we needed to get it done. Though we had to purchase fifty-two gallons of Super Deck stain, we saved on labor.

The week we began the project was very hot, hotter than normal for our nearly 10,000-foot elevation, and, because the sun is so much more intense that high up in the mountains, we decided to do something about it. Our cabin is located in an isolated spot in the woods, and Sally and I had quickly gotten fed up with the heat while we were working. We did the natural thing to do to gain some relief . . . we peeled off our shirts. And this was how, day after day, we routinely worked on the project (living in a secluded valley has its perks). Anyway, one afternoon when I needed to get down off the ladder to open a fresh can of stain, I glanced over at Mary Belle who'd been watching us in her deck lounger. Lo and behold, there she was, sitting there with a smile as wide as a Cheshire cat in contented abandon . . . topless. She'd found a small way to "join" us, and it made her feel more a part of our work than if we'd put a brush in her hand. Seeing her caused me to give a quick double-take and I broke out laughing. "Hey, Sally!" I called to my co-worker up on the other ladder, "look at your Mom! Don't we all look like three woodland nymphs!"

Sally, like Mary Belle, thought that that was really hilarious, and Grandma remained shirtless until we thought she'd had enough sun exposure for one day. With a frown, she obediently donned her shirt and continued watching us work.

The above is a prime example of how an Alzheimer's patient will tirelessly—and seemingly desperately—search for ways to "attach" herself to another's activity. If having a bare top made Mary Belle have a sense of "being one of the girls," or somehow helping us stain the cabin by dressing (or undressing, as the case may be) like an official member of the staining crew, then it served her purpose well. Indeed it did. It gave her a strong sense of belonging, and she associated it with helping us. Even Sally and I felt a sense of how her act of dressing like us served to unify our "observer" with us (the workers) on the job.

After observing this specific, clinical element of Alzheimer's behavior for over three years, we came to believe that the reality of shadowing is, in truth, generated more from a deep-seated fear of isolation than from the more superficial lack of social graces aspect of the disease. The patient's singular intent isn't vindictively directed toward the sole goal of purposely infringing on another's private space, but, more accurately, to be counted among and perceived as being an *inclusive* member of the household, a group, or one of the girls. It's a *social* element. In reality, the behavior surely is closely connected to, and indicative of, a loss of social respect that's only due to the fact that the patient no longer has the ability to give expected due attention to such thoughts of simple politeness, but, rather more to the point, is more personally concerned with and worried about being left out of things or put in an isolated position—which may have the potential of leaving one with the sense of feeling alone or forgotten about.

Mary Belle wanted so desperately to participate in our activities that she'd often be in firm denial over her physical inability to perform certain strenuous activities and chores. This denial was clearly in evidence when we were out cutting and splitting wood or laying railroad tie stairways. She'd adamantly insist that she could do the labor as well as we could, yet it would be undeniably obvious to any child observer that this eighty-one-year-old woman with a severe heart condition, high blood pressure, and two replaced knees could not lift a railroad tie (even a sawed-off, shortened one), shovel yards and yards of soil, or lift large quartz rocks to construct a raised, terraced rock garden.

When we were actively involved in major projects such as these, we had to continually remind her of her health problems and overall physical condition. After she vehemently denied their existence or that it would *not* in *any* way hamper her ability to help us, we didn't waste time arguing with her over it, but instead, would turn the subject around—away from the negative toward the positive—by one of us saying something like, "Know what, Mary Belle? It'd be a huge help to us if you could sit down on that step and take those long spikes out of the bag so we don't have to." Her eyes lit up like a full moon on a clear, alpine night. "See?" she'd squeal in delight, "I told you I could help!"

Times like those were absolutely golden ones. Pure gold. The shimmering glitter of the heart-warming, emotional gilt floated down around the three of us like sparkles of fairy dust and filled up our hearts with untold caches of treasure, whose value was so great it couldn't be counted.

As I've endeavored to convey, the behavior of shadowing is not a symptomatic behavior meant to drive the caregiver, family, and friends up the wall; it's a soulful cry for companionship. It's simply a bid for reaching out for the preservation of remaining self-worth. It's an act of desperation in which the patient strives to avoid feeling isolated, alone, and left out of things—a striving to hold onto the mental capability that is daily slipping ominously away into some obscure black void of jumbled thoughts, unintelligible words, and sometimes . . . even moments of lucidity.

Wandering

The Alzheimer's behavioral symptom of wandering is the one of those *identifiable* clinical traits that is evidenced in every patient during some stage in his/her disease progression. As pointed out in an earlier statement, some behaviors will make cross-over intrusions into other symptoms. Wandering may cross over into belligerence, loss of cognizance, forgetfulness, and paranoia. Depending on the varied circumstances of a particular Wandering event, it can also touch upon Aggressiveness and Obsessiveness.

Wandering is the behavior of simply "taking off." The patient's activities of pacing and restlessness are not true instances of Wandering. Wandering is actually *leaving the premises*. Wandering means goodbye. It means, "I'm outta here!" and "Adios, Amiga!"

So, what prompts this compelling urge to take off and walk out the door? It could be one of a million various thoughts that quite suddenly come into the patients' minds. Perhaps they think that they need to get to a nonexistent job. Maybe they have an urgent thought that it's time for them to go meet someone or that they're late for a business consultation. They might believe that it's time to go pick up some bread or a newspaper. The reasons for Wandering can be as many as the grains of sand on a moonlit beach. When the thoughts come, the patients go. The patients go as if irresistibly drawn by an invisible magnet that compels them to move toward the delusional destination. Their focus on this singular thought is sharply clear and becomes their single-minded purpose-of-the-moment. This single-mindedness is the sole reason why attempting to return the patient to his/her place of residence is often such a difficult task. It is the sensitive trigger for the Wandering to swiftly shift into explosive, physical combativeness when the patient is being thwarted by another individual, a locked door, or some other means which bars the way.

Wandering is an especially intractable behavior for the caregiver, friend, or family member to handle, due to the fact that its preventive management involves constant awareness of where the patient is *at all times*. The caregivers must be continually monitoring the whereabouts of the patient in order to avoid being caught off-guard and left suddenly realizing, with some trepidation, that their patient has "gone missing." Speaking from experience, I can tell you that a caregiver's heart suddenly plunges down into the stomach when this happens (and it will). Immediately upon realizing that the patient is nowhere around, the caregiver first feels that dreaded sinking sensation just before the panic sets in.

An Alzheimer's patient can possess an amazing new talent—that of being extremely quiet when she/he wishes to be. The afflicted individual can be unexpectedly—amazingly—clever, too. Of course, this latter trait seems to be an incredibly incongruous characteristic associated with this type of disease, yet it's also a typical clinical behavior. So it presents a tricky situation for the caregiver to catch whenever it's evidenced by the patient.

The behavioral symptom of Wandering is an especially critical element of the disease. It's critical because it has the potential of presenting an array of hazardous situations for the afflicted individual. Patients can wander away from the home and become completely lost and disoriented. They can walk into moving street traffic, into unfamiliar neighborhoods, get on buses or subways and, in our case, head into the dark woods.

During this Wandering state of mental fugue they can fall or injure themselves in a number of ways. They most often cannot successfully verbally communicate with other people by correctly telling their name or where they live. They've wandered off without carrying any form of identification with them. This is because their destination is their central focus and they don't distract themselves from that focus by thinking about taking a wallet or purse along with them. They just leave. Consequently, it's an extremely high priority for the caregiver to keep one eye on the patient's whereabouts at all times. This high awareness is very important and, after a while, becomes an acquired skill—it becomes the caregiver's second nature.

Examples

When I mentioned the tricky combination of "silent movement coupled with cleverness," I did so from firsthand experience. One night in late autumn, Mary Belle rose from her chair with purpose. She announced, "I'm going to the bathroom," and . . . silently slipped out the back door.

Suddenly the exterior floodlights illumined a movement beyond the window that attracted my attention and, sprinting from my reading chair, I shouted, "Dammit! Sally! Mary Belle's going up the drive again!"

We both raced toward the door to bring her back. Did she intentionally put one over on us by announcing that she was simply "going to the bathroom"? (More on "shining on" in an upcoming chapter on this specific behavior.) Or did she really intend to go into the bathroom and, forgetting where it was, exit the back door looking for it? In this instance, after we caught up with her and asked her where she thought she was going, she didn't respond with "bathroom." Instead, she bristled and said, "I'm going *home!*" The inflection in her voice made it clear that we were supposed to already know that and, if we didn't, *why* didn't we?

"But this *is* your home, Mary Belle," I reminded her, while helping to guide her back to the cabin.

"It is? That's funny. That's the first I heard of that!"

Sally would reinforce the fact. "Mother, you've been living here in Colorado with Mary and me for over two years now."

"I have? Nobody told *me* that!" Then she stopped dead in her tracks and that all too familiar look of deep suspicion would wash over her face. Her head would tilt up at one of us and her eyes would squint in disbelief. "Are you sure?"

"I'm sure," Sally soothed. "Go look up in your bedroom. All your personal things are in there. We helped you put them there over two years ago."

"You did? Over two years ago?"

"Yes, Mother, over two years ago."

"Oh. Well then . . . what are we doing out here?"

Sally had purposely mentioned her mother's personal items that were in her bedroom in an effort to shift Mary Belle's determined attention away from "wandering away" toward the more productive thought of "returning" home to her own room. It worked. That time.

My computer monitor sits in front of a window overlooking the covered front porch. Beyond is the driveway leading into the woods. There were times when, while working on a book, I'd observe Mary Belle go out the back door and then hear the garden gate open and close. I wouldn't immediately get up to check on her, but rather would watch for her to come into view beyond the window. If I could keep her in my sights, I'd leave her to get some fresh air and take in the natural beauty of the property. Oftentimes she was just out for some exercise and not actually "Wandering" off toward some delusional destination. Those were the times when I'd give her some space and, in turn, it afforded her a small sense of independence—that there was no "babysitter" watching over her every move. Most times when she did that I'd see her walking back down the drive, hear the gate, and take note of her reentry into the house. I didn't let on that I'd been observing her the whole time. Yet, there have been other times when she *hadn't* turned her direction back to the house and Sally or I would have to go retrieve her from where she continued on deeper into the forest, or further up the drive toward the country road.

Latitude. The caregiver gives the patient latitude with certain symptomatic behaviors. A walk around the house for leisure and exercise is fine—an innocuous act—but, a walk up and out the drive should be quickly responded to. Both require the caregiver's utmost awareness and monitoring. Both require the caregiver to maintain a split consciousness—keeping the mind on two things at once.

As previously stated, the need to construct a stairway gate at the top of the landing was necessitated by the increased wandering Mary Belle began doing. Wandering downstairs during all hours of the night was not acceptable. Before we were forced to have the electricity cable brought in, this behavior was not only not acceptable, it was not safe for her because there were no lights to switch on and she'd be fumbling around in the dark. She'd be attempting to let her dog outside at three in the morning; she'd try to go out the back gate and wander up the drive or head through dark woods at 2 A.M.

One midwinter night we found her sitting out in the cold car in her thin nightie and bare feet during a blizzard—fortunately, our dogs alerted us. She could've frozen to death sitting out there. When Sally asked her what she was doing out in the car in the middle of the night, Mary

Belle indignantly responded, "Don't you *know?* I was talking to the nicest man!"

The gate at the top of the stairs was one of the most valuable construction projects we put labor into. Though it caused untold bouts of aggressive combativeness and verbal abuse from Mary Belle, it kept her safe during the night and we could rest, fully assured that she would not go wandering off somewhere while we were asleep. Though the gate prevented her from physically taking off during the night, it did not prevent her from experiencing the sudden, compelling urge to wander.

The behavior of Wandering didn't only happen at home; it happened anywhere she happened to be when the mood arose. We could be out dining in a restaurant and, shortly after being served, she'd get up and begin walking away. When asked if she needed to use the restroom, she would usually respond with something like, "No, I'm going to work" or, "No, I need to go let Molly out."

When we took her down to Cripple Creek for an hour or so of her favorite pastime and she'd sit at a slot machine, she'd get up and wander about the casino looking for a way out, or perhaps she'd be searching for someone in particular whom she believed she was late meeting up with, or maybe she'd be desperately looking around for "where they moved her desk to."

When Mary Belle's relatives came to visit one spring, they had her stay over with them at their hotel for a couple of nights. It gave us a short respite, *and* opened their eyes to her condition. Mary Belle often spoke nonsense to them and even wandered off, supposedly to "get a newspaper."

If we took Mary Belle shopping with us (which was rare because she wanted to go home right after entering the store) we had to keep her with us at all times or she'd say that she wanted to just go sit and rest—then she'd walk directly out the door of the mall.

After one Christmas, Sally drove Mary Belle all the way down to the Penney's store at the mall in Colorado Springs so that her mother could exchange a nightgown she'd received as a holiday gift. She'd bugged and bugged us to do this because "she hated looking at the ugly thing." She'd continually make comments about how mean we were not to take her to exchange her nightie. Finally, the day came, and she was excited about the idea of going shopping.

The minute they walked in the door of the store, Mary Belle announced, "I want to go home."

"But we just got here," Sally reminded her.

"I want to go back home. Now!"

"Don't you want to look for a different gown? Look," Sally said, pointing off to the left, "the lingerie department's right here. We don't even have to walk through the store."

Mary Belle's eyes narrowed. "You are so mean to me. You make me do things I don't want to do. If my *daughter* drove me around *she* wouldn't take me places I didn't want to go to! You really take the cake!"

"Shh, I *am* your daughter. And you're making a scene," Sally whispered. "People are looking. Do you want to exchange your Christmas gift or not?"

"What Christmas gift? Is it Christmas? Oh, who cares." And, heading pell-mell for the door, "I'm going home."

Sally dutifully escorted her mother out the door, tossed the unwanted nightie in the back seat and pointed the car in the direction of home—an hour and a half's drive away. On the way, as they were clipping along the highway, making the ascent up Ute Pass, Mary Belle opened her passenger door and tried to step out. With lightning speed, Sally grabbed her mother's arm while maneuvering the vehicle off onto the shoulder.

With her heart wildly thumping over the disaster they'd just avoided, she turned to her mother. "You can't open the door while the car's moving!"

"You listen here, Mister," Mary Belle warned while point-ing her finger in Sally's face, "*you* don't tell *me* what I can't do!"

"Excuse me? You *can't* open a *door* when the car's *moving*! *Nobody* should ever do that. And besides, why'd you do that anyway?"

"Do what?"

"Open the car door."

"I was going to go to the bathroom."

"All you had to do was tell me and I would've pulled into a place with a restroom." Sally merged back into traffic. "I'll stop at the next available bathroom so you can use it."

"Oh, so now you want to make me go to the bathroom when I don't even have to go. Aren't you something."

"You said you needed to use the bathroom."

"Liar."

"You *said* that you opened the car door because you were going to go to the bathroom."

"That's the first I heard of that!"

"Mother, do you or don't you have to use a restroom?"

"No."

One night, when Sally was having a private conversation on the telephone with her brother, Tony, and she was keep-ing him apprised of their mother's deteriorating mental state, Mary Belle became exceedingly agitated over not being able to go down into the basement to hear what Sally was saying. Mary Belle paced and paced before the basement door while wringing her hands in a growing state of woe.

"Mary Belle," I said, "Sally needs privacy when she's talk-ing on the phone."

"But I want to talk to him!"

"You will. Sally will hand you the phone when she's done."

"I want to talk to him *Now!*"

"Well, Mary Belle, Sally and Tony aren't finished with their conversation. You need to wait until they're done.

Then, you can talk to him for as long as you want. You know he always wants to talk to you when he calls. Just wait a few more minutes and you can have the phone."

Pacing.

Hands wringing.

"I want to talk *now!*"

"It'll only be a couple more minutes, Mary Belle. Look!" I exclaimed, going for the nearest distraction. "There's a really good movie starting. Why don't you come watch it while you're waiting."

Suddenly I was speared with a glaring evil eye look; she still wouldn't be deterred from her single-minded mission.

I ignored her demeanor and tried again. "See, Mary Belle? Come look! Isn't this actor one of your favorites?"

With arms flying in dramatic animation. *"You* look, Dummy! I don't *care* about that! I want to talk to Tony *now!"*

One. Two. Three. Four. Counting to ten.

"Well, you have to give them some privacy," I calmly said again. "Everyone deserves to have privacy when they're on the phone. Give them time to say all they want to say to one another. I'm sure they'll be done soon. Sally never forgets to give you the phone when she's done talking to Tony."

I wasn't having any fun riding this verbal merry-go-round she'd pulled me onto, so I made an attempt to stop the ride. I didn't want to play anymore. I jumped off and went to sit on the love seat where I pretended to be overly enthused about the beginning of the movie. Maybe, if she saw how engrossed I was, it would draw her attention to the television screen and divert her attention from the phone.

It didn't work.

From the kitchen I heard an exaggerated sigh and then the cabin shook as the back door slammed with the sound of explosive thunder. In a flash she was striding as fast as she could up the drive—in the dark because we hadn't turned the floodlights on yet. I raced to flip on both front and back switches and then shouted down to Sally. "Mary Belle's trying to run up the drive!" Sally told Tony she'd call him right back and we both went after the irate grandma.

"What're you doing?" Sally asked, after we'd caught up with her.

"Leaving!" she spat.

"Leaving for where?" I asked.

"Anywhere but here! I'm going where I can talk on the phone when I want!"

It didn't take a neurosurgeon to recognize when a situation had escalated into a combative level of behavior. Sally and I nonchalantly positioned ourselves on either side of Mary Belle. This was not going to be an easy incident to reverse.

"Mary Belle," I began, "there's nowhere else to go but here. This is your home."

"Not anymore, it's not!" And she put her palms up as if to warn us away from her, as if to dare us to touch her.

Gently, Sally placed her hand on her mother's elbow in an effort to guide her back down the drive. "C'mon, mother, it's chilly out here. Let's get back into the house."

Jerking her arms out of Sally's grip, she shouted, "Don't *touch* me! I'm *leaving!*"

The situation was not good.

"Mary Belle," I tried, "Tony's waiting to talk to you."

She looked around. "Liar. He's not here."

I pointed to the cabin. "He's down at the house, on the phone."

"Liar."

"Mother," Sally coolly said, "there's no place to go but here. If you don't want to stay here anymore, there's no other place to go to but a nursing home. Do you want to go to a nursing home?"

Mary Belle had gotten herself so worked up that she was actually spitting along with her words. "I can go live with *family*," she replied. "*Family* will take care of me, *family* will let me talk on the phone when I want to!"

Not quite able to ignore the fact that she *was* family, Sally repeated her former statement with calm and an added a twist at the end. "A nursing home is your only alternative other than being here. Do you want to go live in a nursing home, mother?"

"*Yes*! *They'll* let me talk to my son!"

We each reached for Mary Belle's arms at the same time while Sally took the verbal cue. "Okay, mother, let's go inside and we'll help you pack."

"You got that right!" she sputtered, letting us help her back down the uneven, gravel-strewn drive.

Once inside the house, Mary Belle turned on us again. "I will *not* live in a nursing home. Do you hear me? You will not *put* me in one, either!" And with those proclamations given, she strode into the living room and gave her full attention to the television. "I like that actor," she smiled up at us. "He's so good."

"You'll love this movie, Mary Belle," I said, while Sally returned to the basement to call her anxiously waiting brother back. When she was finished detailing the latest incident, the phone was brought up to Mary Belle. "Mom, do you want to talk to Tony now?"

"Oh! Did he call, dear? Yes, thank you, honey."

Event over.

Over and out.

Forgotten.

The act of "taking off" like this incident is a clinically recognized facet of the wandering syndrome associated with Alzheimer's. The patient will suddenly become frustrated, angered, or belligerent over some altercation or event (real or delusional), and simply decide that *leaving the situation* is the only way to handle it. Psychologically speaking, this behavioral response is called escapism. Escapism is a commonly known psychological mechanism in society whereby one chooses the easier route out—one "escapes" the situation rather than having to personally deal with it in a responsible, head-on manner. You don't have to have Alzheimer's to use this imagined "back door" as a way out of undesirable situations. However, there's one big difference between the general public using this means of escape and an Alzheimer's patient using it—as evidenced through the above recounted incident, the patient, more often than not, completely *forgets* why he/she was attempting to "escape" in the first place.

Wandering to anywhere and everywhere, leaving for urgent destinations unknown, and "taking off" in order to escape a situation are common occurrences with those suffering from Alzheimer's disease. Finding out the patient's reason for each specific event is the master key to resolving said situation without the specific incident developing into one of greater emotionality and physical combativeness.

The caregiver learns to use the patient's reasoning as a psychological tool to smoothly reverse course and return the individual home. Once there, the patient can usually be quickly distracted and the entire event, if not completely forgotten by the patient, ends up being one of lesser consequence and, therefore, more easily managed.

First Response Denial

The symptom of First Response Denial is probably the one element of Alzheimer's disease that is most like the behavior of a small child. Even when you catch the child's hand deep down inside the cookie jar, the youngster will firmly deny that she/he was trying to take a cookie. So, too, do the Alzheimer's-afflicted adults have the continual tendency for using denial as their first behavioral response, to avoid owning up to mean-spirited or false statements made and misdeeds done. This denial issues forth with lightning speed when confronted and no amount of rationale (or incontrovertible proof) will alter the patient's determined position of adamantly declared innocence. Like the small child, the commonly heard response to being caught doing something will be similar to, "Not me! No, I didn't do it. It sure wasn't me!"

For whatever reasons—which are only known by the Alzheimer's patients themselves—they will rarely take any form of personal responsibility for their actions. Culpability is not something they're readily prepared to recognize and claim as their own, no matter how strong and obvious the evidence may be for their guilt. And, like the small child, they will behave in a correspondingly indignant manner when questioned. Anger may result, crocodile tears may accompany the denial, animated frustration may be in evidence, or dramatized resentment over being accused can often result in the patient resorting to name-calling—especially "liar."

Is this denial caused by the simple lack of memory of the incident in question? Or could it be an as yet unrecognized natural psychological mechanism of the disease that develops as an offshoot off one of the main clinical symptoms? Or is it merely a desire to remain blameless in all things? From what we've observed, the reason for this behavior would appear to be the latter, for growing evidence seems to be pointing to a psychological ploy for the patient to be perceived as "one who is the epitome of innocence."

Examples

We'd all be sitting around in the living room in the evening and Mary Belle would keep falling forward in her chair fast asleep and snoring; her glasses would be hanging down off one ear. I'd say, "Mary Belle, wake up. If you sleep now you won't be able to sleep tonight."

She'd awaken, straighten up, and look over at me with the glasses still hanging down askew in front of her face. "Oh, I wasn't sleeping."

"Yes, you were. You were snoring."

"No, I was reading."

"Where's your book?"

"Right here," she'd say, still trying to continue the ruse by reaching for the book or magazine that wasn't there. "Oh, it must've fallen on the floor."

At this point I wouldn't push further because she well knew that her game was up. Half an hour later we might witness the same type of scenario after Sally woke her mother up again. We didn't let her sleep all evening in her chair because, if we did, we all paid for it later on during the night when she was up at 2 A.M., kicking at the gate to go to work.

Therefore, for all concerned, it was far more productive to keep her awake, so that she could get a good night's sleep; otherwise the cycle of her body's clock would be thrown off and that, in itself, could generate a whole new array of additional problems.

When the seven pages of my book research notes were ripped out of the notepad and subsequently well hidden, Mary Belle adamantly denied touching them. She even went as far as claiming that she hadn't even seen them. Yet they were right on top of my desk when Sally and I left for an appointment and, when we returned from town, they were gone.

Since Mary Belle had the habit of riffling through our personal papers while we were out of sight, it was all too obvious that she'd been at it again. Sally approached her mother about the notes that had mysteriously vanished during our short absence from the cabin.

"Mother? Where'd you put the pages?"

"Pages? What pages?"

Sally stood before my desk and tapped her finger on the surface. "The ones that were attached to this notepad."

"I don't know what you're talking about. I never touched anything."

While I was already frantically searching Mary Belle's room for my research work, Sally was growing more exasperated by the minute. She sighed. "Look, Mother, you were the only person in the house while we were gone. The pages were there when we left and gone when we got back home. You were the only one who could've taken them. You were the only one because you were the only one *in the house*."

Mary Belle made an Oscar-winning show of innocently looking around her person. Her gaze then lowered to the floor where the dogs were quietly sitting and cocking their heads from one person to another as they listened to the lively interaction. "Maybe those kids took them," Mary Belle offered as her possible solution to the puzzling situation.

"What kids? Mother, there're no children in this house."

"You know . . . the *kids!*" she repeated, pointing down to the dogs. "Kids are always doing things they shouldn't. They're always taking things or messing in other people's stuff."

"You mean the dogs? Are you trying to tell me that the *dogs* took Mary's notes?"

"Well," Mary Belle sighed, "they must have because I surely didn't."

"Oh, Mother, that's the most ridiculous thing you've ever come up with." Sally looked out the window, then back at her mother. "Let's just suppose you did take them . . ."

"I didn't!"

"I said, let's just *suppose* you did."

"You mean like a game?"

"Yeah, like a game. If you *had* taken papers from Mary's desk, where do you think you would've hidden them?"

"Well, I don't know. Let's go look for them if they're missing."

And though we tore the house apart, we never found those seven pages of important research papers that had taken me a week to compile.

A standard response Mary Belle would utilize as an underscore for her denial was this, "Well! That's the *first* I heard of *that!*"; or, "Nobody ever *told* me *that* before!" These were used whenever we caught her sneaking some of her meal to her dog and had to remind her that the vet said the animal was overweight.

The habit of sneaking food to her dog really irritated us because the poor animal needed to lose weight and we'd been taking the extra effort to closely watch what she ate. And, for the dog's sake, as much as for Mary Belle's need for good nutrition, we wanted to be sure Molly wasn't being fed table scraps off the plate meant for Sally's mother to eat.

I'd catch her slipping Molly a huge piece of meatloaf or roast beef from her dinner plate.

First Response Denial

"Mary Belle! Do *not* feed that dog! The vet said it's *bad* for her *heart!*" I reminded her.

"Well!" she exclaimed with a hard glare at me. "That's a likely story because that's the first I ever heard of that!"

No amount of convincing would make her believe otherwise, yet we had to remind her of this fact on an average of three or four times a day, whenever she attempted to sneak Molly some of her meal or some juicy morsel she'd hidden in one of her pockets. By saying that she "never heard that before" or "nobody told me that" she used a mechanism of denial—it served to distance her from being the culpable party, and would naturally preclude her from "having knowledge." So she denied ever having had that knowledge in the first place to avoid responsibility and the consequent guilt it would bring upon herself.

One good example of this first response denial that we witnessed on a routine basis was when one of us would remind her that it was time to take a shower.

"Mary Belle," I'd say, "it's been almost five days since you've had a shower. Let's take care of that today, okay?"

She'd release an exasperated sigh. A smirk full of doubt and disbelief would twist her mouth. "Oh no, no, no. It hasn't been that long."

"Mother," Sally would interject, "are you calling Mary a liar?"

"No, it just hasn't been that long. She's mistaken, that's all."

So then I would have to show her the calendar where we marked the date of her last bathing day. "See, Mary Belle? It was last Wednesday. C'mon, I'll go up and set the shower for you."

And with deep grumbling she'd reluctantly follow me up the stairs.

When we first began receiving all manner of angered calls from her sister, who was reading us the riot act over her "abusive" care, and we were consequently forced to listen to what

Mary Belle was actually saying to people over the phone, we asked her why she was saying such ridiculous and mean things to people about us.

"Mother, why are you telling people that you're not getting fed?"

Mother's eyes widened. "Why . . . you fix *wonderful* meals! I wouldn't say anything like that! Where'd you get such an idea? Honey, I'd *never* say anything of the kind."

"But you have, mother. You've told your sisters that we don't feed you. And you've told them that we never take you anywhere, too."

"Oh! I never, ever said *any* of those things. Why, we go *lots* of places."

It never resolved anything trying to confront Mary Belle about the half-truths or complete nonsense she spoke to people because her sense of denial was so strong. Even if we'd had one of her sisters call back and tell her that she did indeed say those things, Mary Belle would come back with, "Oh, I surely don't remember saying anything like that." Falling back on forgetfulness is a handy tool for Alzheimer's patients. To respond with, "I don't remember," works along the same vein as, "nobody told me that." They both serve to remove the individual from taking personal responsibility.

Mary Belle would give away her personal possessions as gifts and then take them back, denying that she ever gave them away in the first place (as if they were stolen from her).

She would sneak food off her plate and surreptitiously slip it into the pocket of her slacks in order to give it to Molly later on. I watched for that.

"Mary Belle, why did you just put that piece of fish in your pocket?"

"What piece of fish?"

"The one in your pocket."

"There's nothing in my pocket!"

And, at some point in time, we have to make her see that her denial isn't going to always work. "Mary Belle," I said, getting up out of my chair and going over to her. Pointing to her pocket, I asked, "What's that, then?"

She looked down. "What's what?"

"What's that bulge in your pocket?"

"Oh, that. That's my Kleenex."

"Your Kleenex is leaking lemon oil through your slacks."

Finally, she knew the game was up. She looked down at the oily stain on her pants and pulled out the fish. With a sheepish grin, she lied once more. "I was saving that for my breakfast tomorrow morning."

"Don't insult my intelligence, Mary Belle. You know you were going to give that to Molly, don't you."

"Well . . . well, she's *starving* in this place! Nobody *feeds* her!"

Another like incident I caught was when she'd finished eating her dinner in front of the television and had left one good-sized chunk of tender meat on her plate. She made a big show of sighing and smiling wide at us. "That was a great dinner. Oh boy, I can't eat another bite."

I offered to take her plate away for her.

"Oh no, I can do that." She then got up and took her plate into the kitchen.

I followed her.

When she set the plate on the counter, the chunk of meat was missing. Her arm was down at her side, fingers curled around something.

"Mary Belle," I asked, "what do you have in your hand?"

She boldly raised her hand and proudly splayed her fingers before my nose. "Nothing."

"The *other* hand."

Slowly she raised the hand and uncurled the fingers. She made a joke of it. "Oh you, you're too smart. You caught me."

I didn't think it was particularly funny. "That's not the point, Mary Belle. You know what the vet said. Why do we

185

have to keep telling you that it's really important for Molly to lose some weight? Sally cooks good meals for you, Mary Belle. *You're* the one who's supposed to be eating them, not your dog."

"Well, okay," she acquiesced. "I didn't know. People need to tell me these things."

Mary Belle has done the same with breakfast sausage that she's slipped into her pocket tissue. Or she'd be eating and I'd see her nonchalantly push food off the edge of her plate for Molly, pretending she'd accidentally dropped it. We tried all sorts of possible solutions to this problem, even putting Molly outside in the yard during mealtimes, but Mary Belle became so agitated over this particular resolution attempt that she refused to eat altogether unless her dog was in the house with her. It was an ongoing battle we had to fight— one meal at a time. Yet every time it happened again, denial was the same response when caught with the goods.

Mary Belle would frequently speak ill of people. She'd say unkind and mean-spirited things about them, yet when confronted about a particular statement she made, she'd vehemently deny she ever said such a thing. (This was an example of the "backstabbing" I mentioned earlier.) She would gossip about someone and then, to the person's face, adamantly deny ever having said anything negative about them.

If a relative inquired if she'd been out gambling lately, Mary Belle would laugh, "Oh no, no. I don't do that any-more! *They* never take me *anywhere*." Yet she did do it and loved it. She loved it even though she may have become quickly bored. When she said things like, "They never take me anywhere," I wondered if that sort of statement (and others like it) weren't, in actuality, a bid for sympathy.

If reminded that her dog was let outside five times in the previous half hour, she would deny it and attempt to take Molly out a sixth time.

I caught her unwrapping a piece of cheese and starting to reach down toward Molly with it. The dog's mouth was actually open to receive the luscious morsel. "Mary Belle!" I exclaimed, startling her. "You're not giving that big chunk of cheese to Molly, are you?" She quickly straightened up and shoved the entire piece into her own mouth. "Oh no," she mumbled, "I got it for me. See?" Yet, Mary Belle would normally not get food from the kitchen for herself, only for her "starving" dog.

The "scapegoat" excuse is another technique applied for the purpose of shifting responsibility away from oneself. One day, I made Mary Belle's bed four times. Each time I went into her room and found the bed completely stripped, I asked her why she kept doing that.

"He said it needed to be changed," came one reply.

"Mary Belle," I reminded, "there are no *he's* in this house, so how can *he* say your bed needed changing?"

The rationale behind this went right over her head. "I don't know. That's just what he said, so I did it."

"*Four* times?"

"Four times?" she echoed. "Four times what?"

"You stripped all the sheets off your bed four times today," I said while slipping the case back over the pillow. "This is getting really old, Mary Belle."

"You're getting really old?"

"Yeah, Mary Belle," I sighed. "I'm really getting old."

Two hours later the bed was stripped again. It stayed that way until bedtime.

So the first response denial tendency continues to be an ongoing symptom of the disease which patients effectively utilize as a self-protective measure that shields them from having to shoulder blame and take personal responsibility.

For Sally and me, as caregivers, it had been one of the more difficult aspects to deal with because we were never really certain if Mary Belle truly remembered something or not. Between the things she actually *didn't* remember and the things that it seemed *convenient* to not remember lay a very gray area. Our approach to the situation had been to be as consistent with our responses as possible, which, I believe, led to a more stable environment for Mary Belle. Stability and routine seem to ease the patient's fears and lessen the instances of wandering. But regarding the habitual behavior of denying everything, we would just never know if she was trying to pull a fast one, or if she really didn't remember.

Dissembling or being honest?

That was forever the question.

Delusions

In my trusty *Webster's New Universal Unabridged Dictionary*, "delusion" is defined as a psychiatric term meaning: *a fixed false belief that is resistant to reason or confrontation with actual fact.* Delusional beliefs and ideas are common clinical symptoms of Alzheimer's disease. For these patients, reality shifts and reassembles itself in myriad ever-changing, self-devising patterns. Life is rearranged according to the mood-of-the-moment. Reality is whatever the patients believe it to be, regardless of how things actually are. For these afflicted folks, reality may be more as it is for a small child viewing the world through a turning kaleidoscope that constantly shifts, jumbles, and alters That Which Is. This multifaceted delusion factor is the singular element that makes these shifts and jumbles so personally, uniquely, and undeniably real for the individual. It colors the world in a vast array of altered tints and shades of the field of imagination. It may be present in subtle form as obscure shadows and nebulous ideas or it may be evinced by way of crystal clear and razor sharp imagery, both forms being generated from the mind's own bottomless reservoir of phantasmic fancies to draw from. Though that may sound more like hallucination, the mind is, in this case, forming strong patterns of *belief* that have no foundational historical or current factual basis in the patient's life.

Some of these delusional ideas, when the time and effort are expended to deeply analyze them, can frequently be found to contain a single thread that weaves its way back into a patient's experiential past. Though the mind has twisted and colored this fragile thread with various dyes, it can appear to make some logical sense after following it along some very convoluted trails back to its source.

For example, the caregiver of the female patient who was once an architect may discover that the afflicted woman's delusion in believing she now had a job of "tracing patterns" actually goes back to the design-related work of the patient's former career. The male patient who once was a successful proprietor of a national, furniture outlet chain of stores may exhibit signs of the delusion that he's now a "furniture inspector," or he may have developed a compulsive obsession with furniture polish, buffing equipment, or the exact positioning of the household items of furniture as if "setting up a new display room."

Then there are the delusions that appear to have no logical, connective thread to the patient's former life, occupation, or past experience. These are those that seemingly arise out of the blue or, more appropriately, out of the patient's mental field of rapidly misfiring synapses and the disconnected electrical impulses of his/her neurotransmitters.

For the daily caregiver, patient delusional episodes are the one behavioral symptom that carries the most potential for unpredictability, for the patients may, quite unexpectedly, develop new shifts in their world reality at any given moment in time. What may have been yesterday's delusion will, today, be something altogether different. The caregiver quickly learns to live within an ever-changing soap opera that interchanges principal characters and plot lines on a daily basis. Sometimes the perceptions of roles may shift several times in a day. One day the patient may recognize a family member as her/his daughter and the next day that same patient might believe that that daughter is the beautician come to give a perm or the plumber called to unclog the kitchen drain. In the morning the patient may believe her/his home is a hotel and, by the afternoon, swear that that same home is a friend's house and that the time has come to terminate the visit and go back home. Delusions aren't always static; they can be mutable and shift whenever something within the patient's mind is ignited by some subtle spark that flips the trigger switch to a different delusional course, much like a locomotive roundhouse where the engines are moved onto other track lines leading off in new directions for alternate destinations.

Examples

As mentioned in several earlier examples, Mary Belle appeared to vacillate between two delusional careers that had nothing to do with the accounting job she held in life. One was a worker in a shoe factory, and the other was a teacher in an elementary level school setting. Neither "career" seemed to have an associative thread connected to her actual living history. If we wanted to really stretch this analysis for the purpose of discovering a related element, we'd have to turn to psychological aspects rather than trying to search her past experience.

In dream symbology, *shoes* represent "how one's path in life is traveled." A *shoemaker* (as one working in a shoe factory) connotes "an individual who has the capability of guiding the life paths of others." So, working from her subconscious level of perception, we could stretch her current delusional belief in her career as being a psychological act of desperation to "control one's life" (her life) . . . to *maintain the control Mary Belle realized was being lost or slipping away.* From this we could also deduce that Mary Belle was attempting, on some subconscious level, to hold onto continuing control of her own life, and as many related aspects of it as

she could, including family members, matriarchal positioning, career, mother wisdom, etc.

Likewise, the delusion of being a "teacher" can also be
related to her psychological *need to retain her long-held skills
of communication* and/or *her position as an authority figure.*
Again, in dream symbology, a *teacher* denotes "specific
knowledge and the ability to transfer it." Well, Mary Belle
could no longer successfully verbalize her thoughts. Her
expressed words came out jumbled and had no relation to
the originating thoughts that generated those disassociative
words. Subconsciously, she was desperately seeking a return
to her old self, to her former ability to communicate in precise terms and use correct word associations that accurately
convey her thoughts. This, then, makes sense. Though the
shoe factory job and that of teacher have no physical relation to her former life career, they do have a psychological
connection to the situation she found herself caught in.

So what we observed happening was the patient's specific *need* manifesting in the form of symbology.

Mary Belle would kick at the stair gate at 2 A.M., in a fran-
tic effort to get to her school job. She would wander out of the
house with a determined stride as she took off to meet the man
who was going to drive her to her factory job. These "career"
incidents happened, on average, eight to ten times a week.

An imaginary career was not the only delusion we witnessed. Once, her adamantly expressed reason to refuse her
dinner was because, "The doctor told me not to eat!" This
went on for several days, and Sally finally said she was going
to call the doctor to prove that he never said such a thing.
Mary Belle didn't want to talk to the doctor and, perhaps, be
scolded, so she relented and resumed eating.

Frequently, she'd sit all day and cry, just sob and wring
her hands. Sometimes it was quite impossible to elicit a clear
reason from her for the behavior; other times the reason was
a delusional belief. One such mistaken belief was that we

were going to put her dog down. All the reassurance in the world would not change her mind about this. All our various attempts to distract her mind from the thought failed. We even showed her the calendar where I'd noted her dog's next vet appointment for its annual shots. Nothing we could think of doing convinced her that she was mistaken about the idea. Nothing diverted or weakened her conviction. In this case, we had to let her belief take its natural course and loosen its hold on her as time passed. Later, as her disease progressed, she seemed to believe that her son now had her dog. Molly might be lying at her feet while she was talking to her son, but she would ask him, "How's Molly doing?"

"Mother," he would say, "Molly's with you. She lives with you."

"She is with me? Why, nobody told me that!"

And at the end of their conversation, Mary Belle would again ask how Molly was doing.

More than once, I heard Mary Belle talking to someone in the house. An extensive and animated, one-way conversation was transpiring. She was actually answering questions which I couldn't hear being voiced by another. Thinking she was on the telephone, I went into the other room. She was talking to her dog. Another time she was standing beside her recliner and . . . talking to it as though it were a real person.

We tended to ignore events such as those. Sometimes Mary Belle was in her own world, and to tell her that the dog or the chair couldn't converse with her wouldn't serve any constructive purpose. It'd only agitate her and ignite a defensive posture.

I've mentioned the urinary frequency Mary Belle believed she was afflicted with. She was absolutely convinced that she had a bladder infection and that she was actually having to use the bathroom every fifteen minutes when, in actuality, we noted that she used the restroom far less than either Sally or I did throughout the day. Again, all our attempts, using multiple avenues of reasoning, couldn't help her to see the reality of the situation. We tried everything imaginable to dissuade her from this delusion. We tried everything from giving her a notepad and pencil to make a mark every time she used the bathroom to getting her to come to us to announce when she'd just finished using the restroom. Nothing worked. She couldn't remember to use the notepad, or, she'd go to the opposite extreme by sitting in her chair and, one after the other, fill the papers with marks, for something to do. This delusion went so far that Sally finally had no recourse left other than taking her mother to the doctor for tests. Nothing showed up. No urinary tract infection, no kidney stones, no blood in the urine, and no elevated white blood cell count. Still she insisted that she had the "terrible problem" and "how tired she was getting going to the bathroom all the time." We had to inform her that further tests would involve a hospital visit. That was the singular key to nipping the problem in the bud. No way did she want to ever go to the hospital again and be "put in restraints as before."

One winter evening, Mary Belle went to the back door to let her dog outside before going up to bed. The dog was already up in her bedroom asleep. I was in the kitchen at the time and said, "Mary Belle, don't go outside in your nightie."

"Oh, honey," she smiled, "I just need to let Molly out."

"Molly's already up in bed," I informed.

"No, she's not. She's right here."

Mary Belle extended her hand out for me to see Molly. A *Reader's Digest* magazine was in her hand.

"Mary Belle," I exclaimed in surprise, "that's your magazine!"

"Magazine?" she echoed. Not computing what the term was, she reached again for the backdoor knob.

"Where are you going?"

"To take Molly outside," she repeated, stretching her arm out to show me "Molly" in her hand.

Eventually the situation resolved itself on its own when I let her go outside with the magazine. I stood at the door and watched her toss the magazine onto the walkway stones.

"Molly," she ordered, "go potty. Go on. Go on!"

I remained silent.

She then shook her head in disgust, retrieved the disobedient magazine, and came back inside. "Guess Molly didn't have to go," she finalized. Neither of us said another word about the incident.

Sometimes, she thinks I'm Saint Mary. The first time I heard her call me that, chills ran up my spine. I don't know why I had that reaction, but it just affected me in an adverse way. Though folks have made the comment that "we must be saints to put up with all we do from Mary Belle," hearing the "saint" thing come from her own lips was a little too much for me. I dealt better with her calling me the familiar slob slut, which was more her habit to use. We were not saints, just striving very hard to remain grounded while having to constantly deal with someone living in our home who had a deteriorating form of dementia. I don't know. Did the saints of old ever have to deal with myriad feelings of various forms of false guilt? Did they have moments of self-deprecating doubt when they found their resolve wavering and were additionally assaulted with periods of wonderment over envisioned options? Or were they ever bombarded by incoming mental missiles, loaded with warheads filled to capacity with a destructive sense of futility? Who knows these things? Who really knows what multitudes of hidden thoughts a true saint might have had? One thing we knew for sure was that we were no saints. And to hear Mary Belle call me one was unnerving.

The first time she called me that was after I'd brought a meal up to her room. "Oh, thank you, Saint Mary!" she exclaimed with deep appreciation and heavy gratitude in her voice. "I'm so hungry."

I was so taken aback to hear what she'd called me that the chills took precedence over a response. I made none. I just smiled at her and left the room.

The second time she called me that was one time too many. "Mary Belle," I gently said, "I'm not Saint Mary, I'm just Mary. My name's just Mary."

"Oh no," she insisted, "you're Saint Mary. I know you are."

I went over to her bookcase and picked up her thick and well-used Catholic missal. It held many holy cards between its pages. Flipping through the thin sheets of paper, I searched for a specific card. When I found it, I crossed the room, and handed it to her. "*That's* a Saint Mary," I informed. "See, Mary Belle? That's the Madonna holding baby Jesus." I then pointed to myself. "I'm Mary . . . just Mary. You shouldn't call me saint. I'm just an everyday person just like you. Okay?"

"Oh," was all she said back to me.

With that settled, I left the room with high hopes that the issue was cleared up for her, but a week later my hopes were dashed when she used the name again. It left me just as unsettled as it had the first time I'd heard it.

There came a time when her delusion associated with my alleged "wealthy" financial situation became so outrageously out of hand that I finally resorted to doing something with her that I'd never do with anyone else—I showed her my checkbook balance. It so happened that, at the time, it was just before my quarterly royalty check was due to come in and the huge balance showed a whopping amount of seventy-six dollars.

"See, Mary Belle? Can you read that amount? Does that look like I'm rich?"

She looked at the amount. She took the time to examine the check register, scanning the lines of math above the balance in an effort to ascertain validity for the bottom line. "Well," she huffed, "that doesn't prove anything. You just keep all your money in a savings account. You must think I'm stupid or something. I know you're loaded."

I gave up. I had no other account. I kept a little aside in case of some type of financial emergency, but I had no savings account, no investments like stocks or bonds, or any other type of liquid funds stashed away. Neither did Sally. No amount of explanation or show of proof could convince Mary Belle that I did not have a limitless amount of funds available to me. I even tried the logic of asking her, "If I'm so rich, why do I put myself through the frustration of trying to keep our vehicles from breaking down all the time? Why don't I just go out and buy a brand new one to save myself all the hassle?"

She had a quick answer for that. Smugly she replied, "Because you like your money and don't want to part with it, that's why."

We gave up. Maybe she thought we gave up because she was right. We never stopped having to deal with her delusional belief that she continued to share with all those she spoke to. To be honest, it was one of the more frustrating delusions for us to have to ignore.

There are many more examples of Mary Belle's delusional behavior that I could expand upon, but I want to keep them to a minimum. I'd like to close this section with one final example that was somewhat curious to us.

Frequently, Mary Belle would be up and dressed at three in the morning and banging on the stairway gate until we were awake. The reasoning behind that particular urgency to "get out" was not generated by the usual sudden need to get to her job at the shoe factory or the school. It was because, "He told me to. He told me that it's time to go!" And, we wondered, was she dreaming of someone communicating with her, since this specific "reason" always comes in the early morning hours? Was the "he" she referred to her late husband? Was her late husband communicating with her in her dream state? Could she be somehow getting the message that she would be meeting up with him soon? Was she misinterpreting this possible upcoming "passing" to mean that she had to *physically* leave the house?

We would often hear, "He told me it's time to go." Or, once when she was dozing in her recliner and I awoke her, she mumbled, "I wasn't asleep. I'm real interested in hearing what my husband said he's going to tell me."

Now, I wasn't only amazed at what she'd said, but *how* she'd said it. Mary Belle hadn't spoken that many connective words in one sentence in over eighteen months! She'd been in a deep sleep. Had she been dreaming that her late husband was speaking to her? In her dream state, could she communicate normally? I believe that she could because of the reality of the consciousness. Alzheimer's is a disease of the physical brain, not of the mind itself (the consciousness)—the consciousness that survives death. We believed that Mary Belle, in her sleep state of consciousness, communicated on a disease*less* level with her husband. It would appear that, from what she said to us, she was receiving some nebulous indication that her time here on earth would not be long. Therefore, when she awakened from those particular dreams, she retained the main idea but, with the Alzheimer's affecting her physical brain and altering her thought process, she'd then interpret the "leaving" as a need to "go somewhere" but never was able to tell us exactly *where* that somewhere was.

Whenever this specific incident happened, we gently told her that it wasn't time to go there yet, but we'd let her go when it *was* time. This seemed to greatly appease her and calm the heightened sense of urgency and anxiety she had about that particular journey and the additional associative fear of the possibility of us being a preventative force involved with it.

Hallucinations

The hallucination aspect of Alzheimer's disease doesn't usually manifest itself until the patient has progressed into the latter stages of its development. This clinically recognized behavioral element exemplifies the increased and accelerated deterioration of brain function. Some of these hallucinations appear to be directly associated with the patient's specific delusional thoughts, while others are completely unrelated to such existing mental activities. Some are generated by a particular phobia, some by personal desires, others by instigating circumstances only the patient is aware of.

Unlike the sundowning symptom, hallucinations can present themselves any time of the day. There doesn't appear to be a time frame commonality among Alzheimer's patients evincing hallucinations. The incidents can relate to ongoing delusions or they can arise quite unexpectedly out of the blue. There doesn't appear to be a known impetus that serves as a trigger for the onset of hallucinations. They merely come as they may in a haphazard fashion.

Examples

One crisp, late autumn evening when the three of us were enjoying a homey gathering together in the living room, I was reading in my chair by the front picture window and Sally and Mary Belle were both watching a documentary on television. Suddenly Mary Belle leaned far forward in her chair, pointed with heightened interest to the window, and excitedly asked, "Who are those children, looking in the window?"

With a spark of curiosity, Sally and I naturally looked to the window, then back at Mary Belle.

"What children?" Sally asked.

Still pointing to the window, Mother replied, "Oh! Oh, those little kids out there! Why aren't they home this time of night?"

"There're no little kids out there," Sally said. "There's nobody out there."

Mary Belle looked disgusted and gave us an exasperated look, as though to convey that she thought us blind as bats. "Sure there is. Can't you see them? They're looking in at us. They're watching us. Who are they? Do they live around here? Are they the neighbor children?"

I went to the door and out onto the shadowy covered porch. Peering into the living room at Mary Belle, I said, "Come show us. I don't see any children."

In the soft light of the front porch and with the bright floodlights illuminating the surrounding grounds, she looked all about. She looked and looked. "Well," she eventually sighed, "they've gone now. You were too late. They've all run back home now."

After we'd gone back inside Sally and I attempted to help Mary Belle understand that our cabin sat in the middle of sixty acres of nothing but heavily forested woodlands. No other houses. No people around. No children from neighboring homes. Since it was nighttime, we experimented with the alternate logical reason for her sighting as possibly being caused by the play of the reflection of the interior house lights on the window pane. Nothing we tried elicited the precise representational image of what she'd seen—the vision of several small children on the porch looking in at us.

Over the years that Mary Belle has been with us, she's seen these "children" many times—always at night. And, almost every time she saw them, she'd mutter some motherly comment referencing their "sickly" pallor and that "perhaps they were ill children come seeking her care."

Mary Belle worried over these children. She had no other type of negatively associated emotional reaction to them than that. Their sudden appearance, the incidents of their frequent unexpected visitations never startled or frightened her. They had no connection to the sundowning syndrome of the disease. To her, their night presence at our front porch window simply indicated that their visitations indicated something special—meant just for her since we couldn't seem to see them, too.

Sally and I extensively discussed that specific form of Mary Belle's hallucinatory behavior and reached no conclusive resolution for it, since many extenuating possibilities existed for generating its manifestation.

Another time, Mary Belle came up to me and asked, "Would you tell me who all these people are?"

I immediately responded with my own question. "Which people, Mary Belle? People where?"

"Here. Here in this house. Why is this house so full of people all the time?"

"Where?" I pushed, wishing for more information from her.

Again, the old familiar look of exasperation crossed her face. She began pointing everywhere. "Over there. In the kitchen. Upstairs in your bedroom. In your office. A lot of them interested in your office," she added.

Since I'd been sitting at my computer in the office area when this conversation began, I surreptitiously glanced about me. "Here in the office?"

"Oh, for God's sake," she spat with increasing impatience, "*there*, right *behind* you! Looking over your *shoulder!*"

"What do these people look like, Mary Belle? Do they all look alike? What're they wearing?"

She shook her head. "Clothes! They're wearing their nightwear. They're all *old* people! Why are so many old people here all the time?"

Now, to me, these were extremely interesting questions. Spiritually speaking, I happen to believe in life after death and also the existence of angel-like entities. Could the diminished electrical sparking of the physical brain's synaptic activity sometimes serve to expose those more subtle elements of reality that the consciousness, when normally preoccupied, denies recognizing? Or, are most unable to perceive such subtleties because of narrow-mindedness or a mind closed to greater possibilities? Do all hallucinations of those with diminished brain function actually fall into the category of being true hallucinations, or could it be possible for some of these events to be, at times, generated by a clearer view of finer vibrations and dimensional frequencies?

I think there's a viable possibility here for greater research. Just as, many times, we're surprised to discover that a simple solution to a troubling and persistent problem can seem to come out of the blue only *after* we stop putting so much intense thought into it, so, too, might the same conceptual theory apply when a "shift in sight" or awareness results from a state of diminished brain functioning that effortlessly places less focus on the myriad inconsequential details of reality and, instead, allows the mind to "rest in the finer sublime" elements of that same world reality. A mind clogged with details, strong opinions, and misperceptions can often miss seeing the forest for the trees. A mind not cluttered with a multitude of details can see much further, perhaps can see what's right in front of it to perceive and marvel at.

The way I see it, the verdict is still out on whether or not every single hallucinatory event that an Alzheimer's patient experiences can, out-of-hand, be classified as a true hallucination. Though they would initially appear to be so on the surface, I think that there's room here for greater speculation and wiser, investigation of a broader scope into alternate causes.

On the blustery winter night when Sally discovered Mary Belle out in the car, what "man" was her mother supposedly having a conversation with? We know that she didn't perceive the stranger to be her deceased husband, because she referred to him as "the nicest *man*," as though he was someone unfamiliar to her. If she'd recognized him as her husband she would've called him Rudy. Could he be a physical manifestation of some spiritual type of guardian force, keeping her out of the snowfall, keeping her from wandering all the way up the drive or through the dense woodlands? We can speculate about this concept all we want, we can pick it apart and analyze it until we're blue in the face and dizzy from going around in mental circles, yet still come away not being absolutely certain what actually transpired that night. It may have been an experience with a real guardian angel in the form of a "nicest man" or it may have been merely a hallucinatory figment of Mary Belle's increasingly creative imagination. We don't discount the possibility of the man being a guardian angel, for stranger things have happened in this world of ours. And to entirely discount the spiritual aspect of it is to have a myopic view of life.

One autumn day, when Sally and I had been gone from the cabin for an hour or so, we returned to an excitedly animated Mary Belle.

"Oh!" she exclaimed, "I had visitors!"

This is not what we wanted to hear when we returned from somewhere.

Sally inquired, "Who came while we were gone?"

"Three men came."

"Did they come in a car? Did they come down the drive?"

"No, they came up from the valley out front. They just walked up here."

This was curious because normally a visitor would naturally arrive at our place from the driveway. It's the only access off the road. To hear that these "visitors" walked up to the cabin from the valley below was very unusual. There is a cabin at the top of our forested ridge, where our property borders, that is owned by some brothers. It was possible that they'd been out on their land that extended down into the valley the same as ours did. Perhaps they'd walked up to pay a visit since we'd never formally met each other. It was a possible explanation.

Sally continued her questioning. "Did you let them in?"

"Oh, no, we talked outside. We had a nice long talk."

And that's the extent of information we could extract from her. Who the men actually were, or if they were even real is still in question to this day. Our neighbors had never come by during the five years that we have lived here. Why would they happen by on the one day we weren't home? We decided that it wasn't them. We concluded that it was nobody at all. She'd been hallucinating people again and having imaginary conversations with them.

One of the reasons that we decided on this was because, whenever Mary Belle had "visitors," they were always of the male gender. She never had lady friends stop by to visit. This was interesting to us, and we discussed the oddity several times without discovering the reason why she continually hallucinated men instead of women.

The same type of event had happened several times. Even if Sally and I ran up to the post office for the mail (five miles away in Cripple Creek) and immediately returned, Mary Belle would say that two men came down the drive in a truck. Other times she'd report that they just looked down at the cabin and then drove back up the drive; sometimes she'd say that she actually spoke to them. Who knows? These, we tend to believe, are hallucinations that are Alzheimer's-specific—those brought on by a situation of being left alone for a short time. They're her way of denying being alone in the house, no matter for how short a time. We've concluded this because, when she recounted the one particular story about the men driving down to the cabin, it had just rained and we saw no fresh tire tracks in the road other than our own.

The first time Mary Belle informed us that some men had been here while we were gone, we were naturally concerned. This concern came from my being an author whose works are read by people the world over. I've received correspondence from readers in foreign countries who've written that they were flying over to the states to find me for the purpose of going out for a cup of coffee and having a long conversation together. When I lived in more accessible residences, I had folks appear at my door, with suitcases in hand, expecting to camp out on my property. And, as with most other authors and public persons, receiving threat letters over the years also comes with the territory.

So when we moved to this current location, we purposely created extra hoops for ourselves to jump through for the purpose of attempting to keep the residence a bit less easy to find. I, like most other folks, prize my solitude and privacy. Because I'm a well-known author, that privacy can become the most valuable treasure to cherish. Therefore, naturally, we were concerned when Mary Belle began voicing her string of tales regarding all these "men" coming to the cabin while we were away. Perhaps one incident may have involved the electric meter reader who drives down and is gone in a wink of an eye. Maybe another time our friendly propane man came to fill the tank and spoke to her for a bit while he went about his work. Yet, we also have the usual incidences of those people who are merely out for a leisurely mountain drive, taking in the magnificent scenery.

These individuals often ignore a No Trespassing sign on a driveway gate, if that driveway looks as inviting to drive down as ours does. There've been times when I've been out gardening or reading in my chair by the window and have seen a vehicle slowly come down the narrow dirt drive, make a U-turn at the turnaround, look the place over, then head back up and out—completely innocent and well-intended.

I view these innocuous events as folks simply being curious to see what was at the end of the very interesting road that wound through a sun-dappled forest. Many times, they're out looking for property to buy and, if the raw land that they're looking at is nearby, they're naturally interested in knowing what's around that prospective property they're considering. Although I'm not comfortable with people who disregard a No Trespassing sign that's posted on a driveway gate, I understand the interest (and wisdom) of wanting to see what type of neighbors you might end up having if you bought the nearby property. One day, we had a woman drive down to the cabin and come as far as pulling up to the garden gate. She was looking for her lost dog. Sally spoke with her and, after the lady drove off, she came back in the cabin with a flyer in her hand. It had the dog's photo, the woman's address, and a phone number in case we should spot the dog roaming the woods. It turned out that the lady lived a ways up the road and was visibly awed by our valley view when she saw it. She expressed amazement that she'd never known our property was down here—that it was so concealed and hidden from the road up top. That's the way we'd like to keep it.

One morning after breakfast, Mary Belle was extremely agitated. She kept trying to tell us about "something" upstairs, *something* on the floor in front of my bedroom doorway. (Note: Please keep in mind that all of these recounted quoted conversations between Mary Belle and us were not originally verbalized as simply as you read them. She could not get her words out and it sometimes took as long as a couple of hours' time to understand exactly what she was trying to convey to us. For the sake of this book (saving space and reader frustration) I've written all of her statements as though spoken in normal sentences.

So, Mary Belle was trying very hard to tell us about a "big pile of bloody matter that was on the floor in the hall in front of my bedroom doorway." She was growing increasingly frustrated and agitated that nobody was bothering to clean it up.

Our first thought was not "hallucination," but rather that perhaps one of the dogs had gotten sick or had left some type of bloody stool on the carpet. I pulled a couple of rags from the drawer and got the cleaning disinfectant from beneath the kitchen sink.

Sally went for the portable carpet steamer.

The three of us headed upstairs to check it out.

Mary Belle, close on our heels, was clearly grateful that we were finally going to get rid of the "awful" mess that was "stinking up the house."

When we reached the top of the stairs, Sally and I dubiously looked at one another.

The carpet was spotless. It didn't even need vacuuming.

"Mother, where did you say this mess was?"

Responding to that question as though we were both blind, she jabbed her finger down at the floor in front of my bedroom doorway and replied, "Right there! It's right *there*! Look at that horrible *mess* down there! It's sickening!" Holding her nose, she added, "What's the matter with your noses? Oh!" she exclaimed. "Ohhh! Can't you *smell* it?"

There was nothing there. There was nothing there to see or to smell.

Sally bent down and swept her hand over the carpet.

At that, Mary Belle reacted with instant shock. Releasing a horrified cry at the sight of her daughter putting her bare hand in such a gross pile of matter, her hand went up to her mouth. "Oh God, don't *touch* that stuff!"

"Mother," Sally softly repeated. "There's nothing here. See?" she said, holding up her perfectly clean hand for her mother to examine.

And examine she did. Mary Belle then took a tentative step closer to the offending spot and peered down at the carpet. She looked up at us in absolute, honest amazement. "How'd you clean it up so fast? You did a fine job. It didn't even leave a stain! That bloody stuff should've left a stain, you know."

End of incident.

One minute she was seeing a bloody mess on the floor and, an instant later, she was looking at and perceiving a perfectly clean carpet.

Two things about this hallucinatory incident were interesting to us. One was that her hallucination vanished without us having to go through the feigned action of cleaning up the imaginary mess. You'd think that that would've been necessary to make the created image of it go away. Instead, she *imagined* that we'd cleaned it up so fast that she didn't see us do it. Usually, we had to go through some type of *pantomime* to bring the hallucination to a close.

One such example was when Mary Belle, perceiving her *Reader's Digest* as her dog, attempted to take it outside to do its business. Having her follow through with her intent often served to *dispel* her hallucination and return reality to her world. When she threw the magazine she realized what she'd done; she realized that it was not her dog after all. It took her action of actually putting the magazine out in the yard to bring her perception back into focus. But with the bloody mess incident we didn't have to do a follow-through activity (pretending to clean it up) to bring reality into focus for her and that interested me.

The second interesting aspect to this specific "carpet mess" incident was the additional sense of smell that was also a facet of the hallucination. This event involved two perceptual senses: one optical, the other olfactory.

The psychology behind behavioral events such as hallucinations—what sparks their manifestations, what makes them disappear—is fascinating. There would seem to be no consistency of rationale to serve as a concrete guideline. Sometimes a follow-through pretense action makes them go away and, other times, they disappear on their own. The caregiver keeps a finger on the mental pulse of the patient for cues related to the most effective way to resolve each hallucinatory incident the patient presents.

I've noticed that there can be a fine line between an actual hallucination and simple mental confusion. The time I caught Mary Belle having a conversation with her recliner was not a hallucination. She was not actually "seeing" a human form, but rather was confused and disoriented after walking up to the tall chair back. The act of her believing that the chair was talking back to her was delusional.

When she talks to her dog and is, instead, speaking to and looking down at one of our own dogs, that's not hallucination, that's only mental confusion.

When Mary Belle came into the kitchen while I was doing the dishes and poured out her full glass of grape juice onto the counter, she wasn't hallucinating the counter as being the sink; she was just confused.

When she went into the kitchen for a glass of water and returned to the living room with a fork, that was not indicative of her hallucinating and interpreting a fork as a glass of water, that was plain and simple mental confusion. It's important for the caregiver to make this distinction. It's imperative for clear behavioral understanding and corresponding responsive care.

We witnessed another genuine example of this symptom when Mary Belle "saw" the upstairs bathroom as a "bedroom" and, in the middle of the night, frantically shook the stairway gate in her urgent need of getting down to the lower floor bathroom. After the noise awoke us and we tried convincing her that "the bathroom is right there," she would have none of it, believing only what her eyes told her—that it was a bedroom. She could not be discouraged from her perception and thought we were lying to her—again. After running the faucet water and flushing the toilet for proof, the sounds became the mold that served to reshape her reality. She then entered the bathroom and, before closing the door all the way, peered out at us, with a frown of irritation creasing her forehead, and said, "What are you two doing up? Are you wanting to watch me potty or what?"

With sighs escaping from our lips, we turned our backs on her and tried to forget that our sleep had been disrupted. Frustrating? You bet. But humor goes a long way toward alleviating that frustration. A good sense of humor turns irritation and stress into laughter . . . as long as you do it quietly. You *never* want to give your patient the impression that you're ever laughing at *her* because, in reality, it's the *situations* you find yourself drawn into that can be quite funny, not the *individual* doing the pulling.

Mary Belle would be talking to someone when she was alone in her room. One of us would hear this lively conversation transpiring and go up to see what she was doing.

"Who are you talking to, Mother?"

"The monkey."

Monkey? She had a stuffed monkey in her room.

"Mother, are you talking about your stuffed animal?"

"No, Smarty, I'm talking about that *guy* over there," she said, pointing to the stuffed animal.

"But that's not real, Mother. It's not a guy. It's a toy monkey. It's only made of fabric and can't talk. You can't carry on a conversation with that." Sally then picked up the monkey and showed it to her mother. "See?" she said, gently tossing it up and down in her hands. "It's just a toy, Mom. It's not alive. It's made of fabric and cotton stuffing inside."

"Lot you know," came the reply. "He's not going to talk to *you*, that's for sure."

So Sally would leave the room and we'd hear the conversation between Mary Belle and the monkey begin in earnest again . . . right where they'd left off.

Another incident was when Mary Belle came downstairs to find us. She was very excited. "Babies!" she announced. "She had babies!"

"She? Who had babies?" I asked.

"They're all over the bedroom. Under my bed!"

"What's under your bed?"

Mary Belle's eyes were sparkling with joy. "Oh! They're so cute! Come see!"

Up we went with Mary Belle right behind us.

Looking about her room we didn't see anything out of the ordinary.

Mary Belle entered and was full of animation. "Aren't they just the cutest? Be careful not to step on any of them," she cautioned.

We didn't see anything out of the ordinary.

"Step on what, mother?"

Mother sighed in exasperation over our seeming stupidity. "On all those tiny *bunnies* hopping around! What in the world are we going to do with all of them?"

"I have an idea," Sally quickly offered. "Let's close the door so the dogs don't get them. Maybe the mama bunny will gather them all up and take them home where they belong. Then they'll be safe and we won't have to worry about stepping on any of them."

Mary Belle thought that that was a fine idea. She put her finger to her lips to indicate that we needed to be quiet. She motioned us out of her room, checked around the floor, then gently closed the door. "Hope that mama can get them all off my bed."

I smiled at her. "Oh, I'm sure she will. I'm sure she knows exactly how many babies she has. She won't leave a single one behind. You'll see. She'll be a good mama."

And so the three of us tiptoed down the stairs and I turned the television on in the living room to distract her attention from the bunnies. Mary Belle became interested in an old Ginger Rogers movie.

Diversion. Mental diversion.

Sally and I would not mention the baby bunnies again but, after Mary Belle climbed the stairs to retire for the night, we heard her comment to herself after entering the room. "Good mama. You got them all."

We just looked at one another and smiled. Mary Belle no longer had the actual visual hallucination, but she had retained the memory of it.

Psychiatrists and psychologists will attempt to refrain from playing into a patient's hallucination or delusion during therapy. This is due to the fact that these professionals are treating patients who have the potential to gain their mental health back at some point down the road. The patient with Alzheimer's is not going to see a reversal of the disease until such time as medical research develops a cure. This form of dementia only increases in severity as time passes. With most incidents of these people's delusions and hallucinations, there is no success gained by using logic or conversational reasoning to untangle the patient's web of shifted reality. Therefore, they are oftentimes more readily resolved by playing into them, instead of bucking them with logic that will only be met with patient denial, increased agitation, or conflict.

Shining On

The behavioral characteristic of Shining On is associated with "spoofing" others in a manipulative manner for self-serving reasons. Lying, use of fabrication as a means of extricating oneself from responsibility or blame, being underhanded and sneaky, knowing which of the caregiver's buttons to push and making frequent use of that knowledge, having an apparent selective memory when it's convenient to suit a particular situation or is expedient to do so, appearing to possess a certain high level of cleverness in the more lucid states—all of these present a never-ending game the caregiver doesn't want to play, yet finds participation mandatory in order to provide good care.

Shining on isn't an officially recognized clinical symptom of Alzheimer's, yet, through our own experience and in talking with other caregivers, we see it consistently happening with our own patient and with the patients of others. If you research the disease by studying the available reference books on the subject, you'll discover that symptomatic behavior will be widely varied from patient to patient. Some behavioral characteristics will have commonality in all the books while completely different symptoms will be detailed in other related volumes. The reference books appear to have come up with different "official" numbers of stages for this disease. Some list four main stages while others may define as many as eight or nine, depending on how finely the author categorizes the symptoms into separate behaviors.

Shining on fits into this concept of discriminatory reporting on the disease. Many caregivers will quickly recognize this symptom and others will say that they've witnessed little or no sign of it at all. Since Sally and I have personally seen strong evidence of this specific behavior and some other caregivers have too, I would be remiss to exclude it from this material.

Examples

The fact that Mary Belle attempted to sneak food to her dog would appear to point to the fact that she well knew and fully understood that she was not supposed to do that. When she was caught doing it and she responded with the familiar refrain of, "Nobody told me," or "That's the first time I heard of that," she was knowingly using the convenient guise of ignorance as her escape route from shouldering blame and personal responsibility for her actions. Those responses were her way of shifting culpability from herself. If we didn't hear one of those excuses, we'd hear, "I forgot." Yet, why would she be trying to *sneak* Molly the food if she'd "forgotten" that she wasn't supposed to feed her in the first place? The rationale of her excuse didn't fit. Yet, it certainly fits the rationale associated with the shining on behavior.

In previous chapter examples, I wrote about how Mary Belle would not eat unless her food was prepared by one of us, and we set the plate on her lap before the television. Even if she came to us while we were extremely busy, such as being in the middle of a construction project that we couldn't leave, and asked, "Are you going to feed me?" and we responded with, "We can't stop what we're doing right now, Mary Belle. You go get yourself whatever you want to eat," she'd huff away and go sit back down to wait for us to get her food. Yet every time she thought we were both gone from the house, she'd get into the refrigerator and cupboards to help herself . . . and, of course, feed her dog, too.

One example of this was when Sally drove away to attend to errands in Cripple Creek and I was studying some research material at the computer desk. I was sitting at the high-back, swivel chair facing out toward the window, and she probably couldn't see me there. She didn't even suspect that there was a possibility of me still being in the house, believing that I'd gone with her daughter. Behind me, in the kitchen, I heard her tell Molly, "*Now* we can *eat!*" as she got into the refrigerator, took out the platter of baked chicken, and eagerly began feeding herself and the dog. Even if she'd only whispered to her dog, I'd have heard her because, from my computer located at the front of the house to the back door where the refrigerator is, is only thirty feet. It's a small place.

I swiveled around in my chair.

It squeaked.

The look on her face when she turned toward the sound said it all. She was quite shocked to see me sitting there. I'd caught her handing Molly food. Her face flushed with guilt.

"What're you doing, Mary Belle?" I nonchalantly asked.

"I'm eating," she mumbled with her mouth full. "I was hungry."

"Looks like you're feeding Molly."

"Oh no," she said, glancing down, watching Molly noisily chew up the big chunk of chicken breast at her feet.

I didn't think I had to say any more and, swinging back around in the chair, returned to my work.

Mary Belle, too flustered to put away the platter, quickly left the kitchen.

What was so interesting about that particular incident was that she was feeding only Molly and none of our own small dogs that were patiently sitting around Molly and waiting their turn to be handed a tasty morsel. I've watched

Mary Belle go over to the dog bowl while my Keeshond, Cheyenne, was eating from it and take the bowl away from her. Mary Belle then placed the bowl down directly in front of Molly. She had done this so often that I finally had to resort to keeping the dog bowl up on the counter and, several times a day, put it down and call all the dogs to come and eat. The dry dog food we buy is high in nutrition and low in fat; therefore, we've always kept it out all day for our dogs to munch on whenever they wanted, and we'd never experienced any overweight problems with them. Now that Mary Belle believed that her dog was starving, she would take the bowl away from the other dogs and set it down in front of Molly. Then, if one of our dogs should make an attempt to eat from it, Mary Belle would scold it and push the confused and disappointed animal away with her foot.

This behavior was not acceptable to us, because it disrupted the routine that our own animals had become accustomed to. Some of Mary Belle's actions were seriously affecting our animals and their behavior. We observed how many of Mary Belle's behavioral characteristics associated with the disease, such as her screaming during the night, her physical combativeness, her negative attitude, and quickness to argue were exhibited traits that greatly upset the sensitive animals. Consequently, our dogs began to react to these aggressive behaviors in a variety of ways. Due to Mary Belle's belief that she had to be constantly disciplining our dogs (always for no valid reason) and her continual removal of the dog dish from beneath Cheyenne's nose, my dear Keeshond eventually developed the "rage syndrome" and we had to have her put to sleep because we could no longer trust her response to Mary Belle as being an understanding one. That was a very sad day for me. The other dogs (our four Yorkies) developed a nervous wariness and would avoid Mary Belle whenever possible, because she was so unpredictable and caused them much confusion. As a result of Mary Belle's behavior, the Yorkies began having more accidents in the house. Animals are extremely sensitive to people's moods and are acutely attuned to their emotional states. This fact was never so clearly proven as after Mary Belle came to live with us, and our pets responded correspondingly to her aggressiveness.

One evening, while the three of us were watching television in the living room during dinner, Mary Belle kept surreptitiously looking over at me and giving me side glances. She knew that I kept watch during mealtime when Molly was sitting at her feet and pawing at her leg in attempts to beg for some food from her plate. Though I wasn't so obvious that I actually stared at her while she was eating, I would keep a peripheral awareness of whether or not she was slipping Molly some of her meal.

This time Mary Belle suddenly pointed out the window beside me. "Oh, look!" she excitedly exclaimed, expecting me to immediately respond by falling for her ruse. She then swiftly grabbed a piece of meat from her plate and dropped it at her feet in front of Molly's paws.

She hadn't planned on me *not* looking out the window.

"Mary Belle!" I said. "*Don't* feed your *dog*! The vet said not to."

"Oh," came the innocent reply. "Nobody told me that."

Of course, by now the dog already had her food, and Mary Belle had been satisfied that Molly wouldn't starve that night. Mary Belle's mission had been successfully accomplished.

So, then, if nobody told her that she wasn't supposed to feed her dog morsels from her dinner plate, why'd she try to play such a four-year-old child's trick for the purpose of distracting my attention away from her intended act?

Shining on?

Mary Belle reached a point in the progression of her disease where she absolutely despised bathing. She would never initiate the activity. When one of us reminded her that it was time to take a shower, she'd vehemently deny that she needed one or else she'd refuse to believe how many days it'd been since her last one was taken. Yet . . . when her daughter Judy was coming out to Colorado to visit us, Mary Belle wanted to take a shower every day for a week before the arrival date. So what was with the refusal to bathe on a regular basis? Shining us on? Exercising her right as the elder in the home to claim greater knowledge than the others? This last was a frequently used behavior.

We also noticed that Sally's mother appeared to have a selective memory. She would remember the kind and endearing things she'd said about someone but would absolutely deny any of the mean-spirited things she'd said. She claimed denial of them or that she simply "forgot" the offending statements were ever made. True forgetfulness? If so, how can such forgetfulness be so selective as to separate the negative statements from the positive ones? The ones that will boost her self-image from those that will lessen it? Shining on in an effort to remain blameless?

Mary Belle's disease had rapidly progressed in the time she'd been with us. After three years, whenever she wanted to tell us something, she could not seem to effectively verbalize her thoughts in a consecutive arrangement of rational words. Yet, whenever she'd be on the telephone with her other daughter, her words would flow together and complete sentences would follow one another. Could it be possible that the use of an instrument of communication such as a telephone could in some way facilitate an improved method of thought transference from the mind into better verbal skills? Or was her constant, seeming inability to clearly speak with us an "avoidance" of such interaction and a real example of shining on?

Sally, Tony, and I noticed her utilization of yet another psychological ploy that is usually associated with rational and lucid individuals. Mary Belle would sometimes play one sibling against the other. This required planning for such manipulative, mental maneuvering. When it occurred, it was usually motivated by something Judy had said to her. While talking on the phone, Mary Belle might not be able to verbalize the precise word she was wanting to voice and Judy would fill in the blank for her mother.

One example of that was when Mary Belle was having difficulty while attempting to say something about Sally and immediately Judy did the "filling-in-the-blanks" thing. She asked, "Sally's *bossy* with you?" And Mary Belle responded with, "Oh, yes! All the time!" Then you get, "Well, mother, if you lived here with me, I wouldn't boss you around."

Mary Belle has, on a number of occasions, tried this same maneuver with her son, Tony. Yet, Tony knew that his sister wouldn't exhibit any type of negative behavior toward their mother, so he quickly stopped her in her tracks when she tried those negative sibling tales with him. He and Sally had extended weekly conversations regarding the various behavioral elements of the disease, which had been increasing in severity and occurrence. They are both intelligent individuals who've come to realize that this particular behavior is instigated by a simple, psychological bid for sympathy.

The interaction between the immediate family members of a loved one with Alzheimer's is critical. This familial aspect is always presented as a major issue in every reference book we've read on the disease. The specific interaction that's most important is that of *supportive reinforcement* given to the family member who's been delegated as the loved one's primary caregiver. When family members participate in a tug of war with one another, with the parent in the middle, not only does this make the caregiver's job much more difficult, but, along the way, everybody suffers the consequences.

As in the previous example, perhaps Mary Belle was going to say something altogether different about Sally, yet she didn't bother to object to the word that was quickly interjected as a "fill-in" for her because, as I've seen her do time and time again, Mary Belle found it too tiring and frustrating to extend the conversation time while people waited for her to finally verbalize the exact word she initially intended. Instead, she'd merely agree with whatever someone else filled in for her, whether that was the correct word she meant to say or not. Though Mary Belle would have the awareness to know that the fill-in word wasn't what she wanted to convey, she'd not take the time to correct it, letting a *negative* or derogatory idea about someone go unchecked, instead.

Friends and family members of Alzheimer's patients need to realize that this goes on. Talking *for* the patient and filling in the difficult-to-express words doesn't always result in accurately communicating what the patient meant to convey. However, we noticed a growing tendency for Mary Belle to play one adult sibling against the other. And, when approached about this behavior by her son or Sally, she'd completely deny she did any such thing and would end up calling them liars. Oftentimes, trying to reason with such a patient is futile and the easiest recourse is to just let the incident pass without adding further complications to the event.

Another time, when Mary Belle saw Sally drive away and thought she was left alone in the house, I came up the basement stairs after putting a laundry load in the washer and caught her red-handed at my desk . . . with a stack of my bills in her hand. She'd been going through them and already had three of them stuffed down in her pants pocket. When she saw me, she literally jumped, her entire face flushed red with embarrassment, and she immediately dropped the envelopes as if they were hot potatoes.

"Mary Belle! What are you doing at my desk? There's nothing of yours there."

"I thought you went with Sally."

"I was down in the basement. What've you got in your pocket?"

"Pocket?" she echoed, looking down at the floor.

"Mary Belle, in your pants pocket!"

She then patted her pocket. "This?"

"Yes. What've you got in there?"

"Oh, nothing."

"Then what's that bulge in there?"

She touched her pocket. "This?"

I nodded. "That."

"Oh. That's just my phone list."

"May I see if you have the right list?"

Finally she sighed with resignation and sheepishly pulled out the scrunched bills.

"Mary Belle," I asked, "what're you doing with my bills?" I held them up. "What were you going to do with them?"

"Bills? Well . . . I don't know."

"Why did you take my bills, Mary Belle? You know that this is my desk. You know that there's nothing of yours on it."

"Well!" came the indignant response. "That's the *first* I ever heard of *that!*"

Yet it was probably at least the hundredth time she'd heard it. So what do you do? Her flushed face reaction to my sudden, unexpected arrival in the room, and her sheepish look over being asked to empty her pocket all pointed to knowledge . . . knowledge that she had indeed realized she'd been caught doing something she *knew* she wasn't supposed to be doing. Her evasive responses to my questions and the final denial statement of, "that's the first I heard of that" all clearly point to the "shining on" behavior.

Sneaking followed by quick denial is an element of this behavioral trait. Logically, if someone truly forgets they're not supposed to do something, if that same individual truly believes that they've never been told not to do something, or that they never heard of it before, they'll have no reason to be surreptitious about doing it—they'll do it right out in the open as if it was the most natural and perfectly allowable activity to perform.

It was evident that Mary Belle always seemed to think that I was in the pickup with Sally every time she drove away from the cabin. This meant that she believed we left her alone. In truth, I rarely accompanied Sally on daily errands for two reasons; one was because we didn't want to leave Mary Belle alone in the house, and the second reason was that we have publishing and our craft business calls coming in. When you're trying to carry on two types of self-employed businesses in your home, you naturally try to be available for related incoming calls. I'm rarely gone and, when I am, it's usually only when the respite caregiver is here to be with Mary Belle. So then, the habit of thinking I was gone with Sally every time she pulled away had been extremely eye-opening for us. If Mary Belle didn't visually see one of us, or hear us moving about, she automatically assumed that we were not home and would immediately begin snooping into our personal papers or getting into the refrigerator to feed her "starving" dog.

This behavior showed us that Mary Belle *did* know that she was not supposed to get into my desk and private papers. It showed us that she *would* get into the refrigerator and kitchen cupboards to get herself (and Molly) something to eat. So the obvious questions are these . . . why didn't she get *herself* something to eat when we were home? Was it because she wanted *us* to get it *for* her? Why didn't she get into my desk when we were home? Was it because she *did* know that she wasn't supposed to? Shining on. That would seem to be the answer to these puzzling queries. Maybe we'll never know, but it sure seemed likely.

Preoccupation with Death

For the Alzheimer's patient, thoughts of death in varied forms are a commonly demonstrated clinical symptom. Even in the more lucid moments, these thoughts persist in a manner the patient associates with personal uselessness. I personally find this interesting because, for the most part, the patients themselves don't normally realize that there is presently no known cure for their condition, that the end stage is a terminal one.

Having written on the subject of spiritual philosophy for nearly two decades, my thoughts on this seeming enigma are naturally interlaced with consideration of spiritual ramifications and related elements. Could it be possible for diminished brain function to heighten an individual's awareness and sensitivity toward the finer realms of reality, whereby the patient's consciousness, relieved from the massive sensory bombardment of external reality, becomes an open receptacle for the more subtle aspects of reality—wherein intuitiveness, prescience, and the language of the spirit are as common to her as the verbal communication of the third dimension? Does consciousness shift to a different—a higher and finer—frequency, in an effort to compensate for the loss of current, real-time cognizance on the touchable, physical level?

The types of behavior related to this typically documented symptom that Sally and I had personally observed in our patient would seem to make this theory far more than a weak, far-reaching, or wildly speculative possibility. Even in those rare non-lucid states, our patient still had a will to die based on altogether different reasons than those of a lucid thinking individual—reasons more closely associated with *joining* the spirit realm rather than directed toward the act of *leaving* the physical. This distinction between the two purposes is telling, because it indicates that in the lucid and the non-lucid mental states, there is a *disparity* in one's underlying reasoning for wanting to die.

Examples

When Mary Belle first came to live with us, this behavioral symptom was not initially in clear evidence. In fact, her entire view of life was quite the contrary, in that she was extremely excited to be living in the natural beauty of the Colorado mountain high country. She'd repeatedly enjoyed sharing happy reminiscences while telling me all about the various Colorado vacation trips she and Rudy had taken the family on when her children were youngsters. They'd camped and had wonderful times in what she called "God's Country."

Later, though, when the disease gained a greater hold on her mind, the "death symptom" began showing up in subtle ways. She would never come right out and state that she wanted to die, but would, instead, make insinuating statements such as, "You don't need me around here," or "Where do you keep your guns?"

As time passed she progressed to the stage of thinking about giving all of her personal possessions away.

One day, when Mary Belle was upstairs in her bedroom, her movements sounded as though she was moving furniture around. Sally went up to find out what her mother was up to.

Seeing that Mary Belle had meticulously made piles, spread all about the room, of blank note pads, paper clips and pens, and clothing, Sally asked, "Mother, what are you doing with all of your things? Why did you make piles everywhere?"

"Oh . . . I'm giving them away," she nonchalantly replied while pointing to each grouping of possessions. "This pile's for Judy. That one over there is for Judy. And this here is for . . . ah, this here's for Judy."

Sally again scanned the various mounds of disparate items. "Mother, you've made a pile of your underwear! Here," she gently offered, reaching for the stack of clothing, "we need to put these back in your drawer."

Mary Belle became instantly agitated with that. "No! Don't touch those! I don't need them anymore!"

A frown furrowed Sally's brows. "Why on earth don't you need your underwear?"

"Because I'm leaving, that's why."

"You're leaving? Where are you going? Won't you still need your lingerie? Your underthings?"

"Not where I'm going, I won't."

Clearly, Mary Belle was in her "preparing to die" mood.

"Oh, for heaven's sake, mother, not this again. You're not going to die," Sally reassured her, while reaching for another pile of possessions to put back where they belonged. "What is *this* supposed to be? Why is your wastebasket on the bed?"

"To give to Judy, stupid."

Sally ignored the name-calling. "You're going to give your trash to her? Mother," she sighed, "you're confused, that's all. Even if you want to give your things away, no one's going to want this old wastebasket." The small plastic bin was replaced on the floor behind the door.

Eventually all the piles were put back where they belonged. Although Mary Belle had made piles of possessions that were not appropriate to give away, the fact remained that she'd been thinking of dying and wished to be certain that her possessions were taken care of and properly dispersed to family members. In this case, it was interesting that nothing was designated for her son or for Sally. In her impaired state of mind she'd thought of nobody but Judy, because Judy was sometimes the only person she remembered being related to. The other times she'd made these piles of belongings they were solely designated to Tony, or to Molly, or to Sally. By now the notarized will she had made while still of sound mind was not a part of her current memory or reality. Now, she was bequeathing her underwear and the entire contents of her wastepaper basket to whomever she could recall at the time. These "remembered" people changed on a daily (sometimes hourly) basis.

When we bought Mary Belle the activity table for her room, she immediately became upset with us when it was delivered to the house. Her agitation over this gift was evident when she began nervously raking her fingers through her hair.

"What's the matter, mother?" Sally inquired. "Don't you like the table?"

"Oh, yes. It's very nice. But I hate to see you waste your money on me like this. I won't be here long enough to use it. Can't you return it and get your money back?"

"Mother, please don't start that dying talk again. We're not returning this. You're going to be with us for a long time. You need a table for you to work your activity projects on."

Mary Belle released a long, drawn out sigh and shook her head. "Thank you. Thank you both for the table." Clearly she didn't believe what her daughter had said regarding her longevity, but also didn't want to make a scene over their difference of opinion.

In one of Mary Belle's more lucid moments which were appearing more and more infrequently, she insisted that Sally take care of a pre-paid cremation arrangement for her. She also talked to one of her close friends from her church back in Shawnee Mission, Kansas, about writing her a scripture eulogy for her own funeral service. The friend was happy to assuage Mary Belle's concern and agreed that it would be taken care of for her.

Several months following those incidents, Mary Belle exhibited suicidal tendencies. Many mornings she'd refuse to accept her proffered medications from Sally, saying, "I'm not taking any more pills. Take them back where you got them."

Sally, feeling as though this was the beginning of a daily rerun, said, "Mother, you have to take these. They keep your blood pressure regulated and help your heart."

Defiantly, her mother replied, "Put them back. I don't want them."

"Why?"

"That's my business, not yours."

"It is my business, mother. Part of my job is to care for you and try to keep you as healthy as possible."

Silence.

"Mother, why won't you take these?"

"Don't play dumb with me. You know why."

"No, I don't. Tell me."

"I'll die sooner if I don't take them."

"No, you won't, because I'll put you in the hospital if you refuse your medication. The doctors will give them to you through an I.V. line or injections."

Mary Belle reached for the pills and took them. "Don't you *ever* put me in a hospital! I will not go to one again! Do you hear me? I do not want to go to a hospital again! No matter *what!* Promise me that you won't take me to a hospital ever again. I have a DNR order, you know."

So the medication was dutifully taken this time. At least three times a week, Sally and her mother repeated the same scenario over morning meds.

Several times a week, Mary Belle would approach Sally and firmly make a declaration. "I'm not going to eat any more."

"Why not?" came the natural response.

"I'm going to starve myself so I'll die sooner."

"Then you'll force me to put you in a hospital, where they'll feed you intravenously. You'll still get your nourishment, and you won't end up starving. So you may as well go ahead and get your nutrients from the meals we fix and enjoy the taste of everything you like to eat at the same time."

Mary Belle would make a face, stick out her tongue at Sally, and turn on her heels. Though she'd keep up this childish behavior for the rest of the day . . . she'd reluctantly eat her meals and let us know that she was doing it against "her better judgement."

Ending one's own life is not the only evidenced behavior of this symptom of being preoccupied with death. Ending the lives of others also comes into play. On the evening of July 20, 1999, when Sally had our empty shotgun out to take to the shop the following day to have it altered, Mary Belle had been in a particularly confused and ornery state of mind. She'd been in the mood all day long due to a stubborn delusional episode. She'd kept trying to tell us about "some man who was in the house with a little toddler." She was extremely agitated over this strange man and boy. She exhibited agitated paranoia that the man was dangerous. Although we kept reassuring her that there was nobody else in the house but us three women, she grew combative over her obsession with the idea.

As I was preoccupied while washing the dinner dishes, I was startled when hearing Sally suddenly shout behind me, *"Mary Belle!* You *give* that to me!"

I spun around to see Sally yank the shotgun out of Mary Belle's hands. Her mother had had it aimed at my back.

My stomach churned. "Oh, my *God,*" I whispered, quickly thanking the Powers That Be that the gun hadn't been loaded.

Sally was furious. "What were you going to do with that, mother?"

Mother appeared nonplussed. Calm. "Well, I don't know. I guess *take care* of everybody before that *man* did. Maybe I was just going to take care of *me.*"

(Important side note: Mary Belle had no access to loaded guns. Sally is a gun collector. We have everything: palm-sized .22's that look like pagers when clipped to one's pocket, larger caliber magnums, to a .7mm hunting rifle. Ever since the first time Mary Belle asked us, "Where do you keep your guns?" our prescient alarms went off, and we took immediate measures to keep all weapons and ammo out of harm's way.)

As the disease progressed, Mary Belle's fascination with death seemed to be more and more associated with "talking" to her deceased husband about the subject of death and dying.

We would have events that quickly turned aggressive and physically combative when we had to prevent her from leaving the house after she repeatedly shouted in our faces, "He *told* me I have to *go!*"; or, "He *said* it's *time* to leave now!" And she'd push us, pummel with her fists, slap faces, kick, bite, and do all in her power to get past us and out the door when this thought (or directive) came over her.

Other incidents involved her waking from a night's sleep or an afternoon nap and relaying a clearly remembered "conversation" she'd had with her deceased husband. "He's going to meet me now. I have to go!"

That is when we had to devote hours to calming her down and convincing her that it was only a dream, that when it was really time for her to go, we wouldn't prevent her from joining Rudy. Mary Belle's dementia made it extremely difficult for her to separate the present, third-dimensional reality from the reality of other dimensions and states of consciousness.

She was misperceiving her dream state reality as being identical to her three-dimensional reality. There appeared to be no evidence of any differentiation between the two. We witnessed this confusion whenever she awakened from a dream state in which she recalled clear communication with her deceased husband. Perhaps he was communing with her. No one can really say for sure. Perhaps he was telling her that they'd be together soon—stranger things have happened. However, when Mary Belle awakened, she thought she had to leave "now." Her interpretation of "leaving" was transferred to the idea of physically leaving the house. Her strongest thought at that time was that she must leave, yet she had absolutely no idea where it was that she must go. She'd try to walk up the drive to accomplish this leaving that she associated with "going to be with Rudy again."

This symptom had deepened into one that included the desire to "do away with others," particularly when the patient's desires were thwarted for some reason. If Mary Belle didn't get what she wanted (usually thwarted desires such as refusing to take her medication or eat her meals) her mood would turn verbally aggressive and she'd begin talking about how she was going to kill us. She'd go on for hours about killing us and, to be honest, one quickly wearies of hearing that sort of morbid talk in one's home, especially coming from a loved one. Although we understood the talk was coming from dementia, it was still distressing to hear so often.

Whether Mary Belle had conversations with her deceased husband, who told her that they'd be together soon, or whether, in her more lucid states, she just didn't want to be a burden to us anymore, the fact remained that thoughts of her own death were clearly never far from the forefront of her mind.

But the thoughts of death turned into a strong, conscious desire to see it actuated. For her caregivers, that resulted in a constant vigil (and battle) to maintain optimum health care against her will. Sally loved her mother. Mary Belle wouldn't have been there if she hadn't. Sally wouldn't have put up with the extreme frustration and frequent verbal and physical abuse such a patient exhibits from the disease if she didn't deeply love her mother. Though Mary Belle wanted to die, both Sally and I saw that she was still experiencing many enjoyable days and reasons to be happy. For Mary Belle there were still reasons to live. Her quality of life was good—better than good. She had family with her. She had her beloved dog with her. We bought her an aquarium for her room, and a parakeet. She had a room of her own and enjoyed full run of the house and grounds (even though we had to monitor her outside ventures). We took her out to dinner, to the beauty shop, and sometimes she'd accompany Sally on her errands about town. She frequently talked to her old friends on the phone. Her sister came to visit her as well as her other children, Tony and Judy. She lived with people who gave consideration and deference to her personal interests and went out of their way to provide ingenious activities to keep her active and make her feel productive. Although there were days when Mary Belle wanted to do nothing more than to sit in her recliner and stare out the front window, she still had a beautiful mountain valley to look at and a multitude of bird varieties and small four-legged critters to watch come feed on the porch. No, her "leaving" time had not yet come.

Reaching the Retaliation Stage

In a previous chapter, I mentioned that our patient would pummel with her fists, slap our faces, bite, and kick. Physical aggression was the beginning of a new stage of actual combativeness that hadn't been exhibited up to that point. Before then, she would only make the "motions" of doing these acts of aggression. Later she followed through and carried them out. Her dementia had made a dramatic turn by, seemingly overnight, suddenly accelerating to the point of her behavior becoming so violent that we quickly learned never to turn our backs on her. Never. It had become a retaliatory behavior, where she exhibited the routine habit of suddenly, without the slightest hint of provocation, striking out with full-blown blows with her fists, digging her nails into one's skin, biting with lightning speed, kicking out, and grabbing at the nearest object to wield as a weapon and swinging it with all the force she could muster. Accompanying this behavior were increased verbal statements expressing her desire and intent to "kill us."

Examples

On the evening of September 26, 1999, while Sally was busy working on her metal sculpture in our basement workshop, I was sitting with Mary Belle up in the living room. She was watching television and I was proofreading through the final copy-edited pages of my *Beyond Earthway* (Pocket Books, 2000) manuscript. While I was busy giving my attention to this, I'd also observed that Mary Belle was becoming more and more agitated as she crisscrossed the room, trying to settle in one chair after the other.

I asked her if anything was wrong.

"I can't seem to get enough breath," she replied. "I'm having some trouble breathing."

Setting my work aside, I guided her over to her recliner and opened the footrest so she could elevate her feet. It was then that I noticed her ankles were more swollen than usual and it sent up a glaring red flag. I removed her shoes and rubbed her back a bit in an attempt to soothe her increasing agitation.

"Ohhh, honey," she sighed, "that's so much better. I can breathe better now."

Although I returned to my place on the love seat, I kept a watchful eye on her. A few minutes later her breathing began sounding congested with rattling noises in the lungs. I put my papers down and went back over to her. She again complained of having difficulty breathing. Recognizing the onset of a physical crisis, I called for Sally, who immediately rushed up the stairs two at a time.

Mary Belle's chest rattle was becoming worse, as was her effort to gain enough air. As Sally tried to assess the situation by asking her mother questions, I knelt beside the chair and stroked Mary Belle's hair. She kept alternating between her wishes by saying that she "wanted to go," to "*please* let her go," but then countered these with, "call a doctor." Sally gave her a nitroglycerin tablet to put beneath her tongue, and we waited with her. We waited to see if the symptoms would subside with the medication, all the while listening to her plead with us to let her go. We told her that she was free to go whenever she wanted, that it was alright.

When the condition didn't look like it was going to significantly improve, and even though Mary Belle had a signed and notarized DNR order, she began asking for a doctor more often than she was asking for us to let her go. Sally's emotions took over, and she called for the ambulance.

When the paramedics arrived, they took readings with their various machines, made a couple of calls, and announced that the patient was experiencing congestive heart failure, which was a completely new medical condition for her. Mary Belle didn't like wearing the oxygen mask and kept trying to yank it off her face. I had to keep telling her to leave it alone, that it was helping her to breathe. The ambulance left with their transport patient an hour later, with Sally tailing it all the way down to the hospital in Colorado Springs.

Because Sally was the only one of us witnessing the rest of the week-long events, she's the one to now take over the narrative of her mother's hospital stay and its ensuing events. The remainder of this chapter is written by Sally herself.

When we arrived at Memorial Hospital the ambulance team didn't waste time expressing their displeasure with me for "following" them all the way down the pass. According to them, I was supposed to just meet them there, not tail them. At that point, the last thing I needed was their chastising attitude. I was upset and worried enough about my mother without having some strangers get in my face as soon as I got out of my car. I'd followed them because I wasn't sure of the hospital's precise location. I'd only been there once to visit a friend after her operation and couldn't recall which roads would be the most direct route. The team seemed to be placated by that reason, and I followed close behind the gurney as it was rolled through the emergency department doors.

The hospital staff quickly descended on both my mother and myself as soon as we entered their domain. IV's and monitors were hooked to her while I was busy giving her medical history. We were in the emergency room almost four hours that night. The first two hours were fairly calm and Mom actually fell asleep while the lab was running its tests. During the time that we were waiting for the results and a procedural decision from a doctor, another emergency patient was rushed through the doors and the team needed to move Mary Belle into another room.

Mother didn't seem to like being moved away from the center of everyone's attention.

Soon after she was situated in the second room, a lab technician cheerfully entered to draw more blood samples. No sooner had he gotten a good vein (no small feat), when mother angrily jerked her arm back, dislodging the needle. Leaning forward, she glared hard at the poor man and hissed, "Damn you!" Quickly recovering from his initial shock at her behavior, he bravely wanted to make another attempt. I assisted him by holding her arm still and he finally left with his prized vial.

Our next visitor was a woman who wanted to hook Mom up to the heart monitor. As soon as she reached out to open mother's gown, Mary Belle grabbed the woman's arm like a human clamp and started trying to gouge her fingernails into the lady's skin. Immediately reacting to this unexpected behavior, I tried to pry Mom's hand off and was promptly bitten for my efforts. Needless to say, the woman speedily exited the room without successfully achieving her intended goal with the heart monitor.

Once in her bed, Mom immediately took the chance to display her newly formed "wounds." She boldly held out her arms that were already full of bruises from the IV's she'd repeatedly pulled out, and scathingly announced to anyone within earshot, "Look at this! Sally *used* to love me, but look at what she's *done* to me!" Those professional personnel who were in attendance knew that I hadn't caused Mary Belle's bruises. They were aghast to hear the patient's claims. My heart ached to hear my own mother accuse me of causing the very bruises that she herself had inflicted upon herself only moments before in the emergency room. And, upon hearing her sobbing accusations, all six of these medical professionals looked in shock at Mary Belle and then, they cast their glances over at me without uttering a word. It was an extremely odd and highly uncomfortable moment, one of many when there are just no words, yet I felt like asking these professionals, "What? Haven't you ever dealt with an Alzheimer's patient before?" But I resisted the urge to voice the question that wanted to spill forth. I held my tongue. I didn't whisper a word. Instead, I left the room with one of the nurses who wanted to take a more in-depth medical history.

It was now going on 3 A.M.

I spoke with the nurse for about half an hour, answering questions about everything from the patient's medical history to her current living conditions. The nurses just couldn't seem to believe that this severely aggressive patient actually lived at home and that Mary and I had not brought in outside help to assist with the management of her difficult Alzheimer's condition.

"How do you do it?" one of them asked in amazement.

"One day at a time," I replied.

"Do you keep her sedated?" another inquired with high interest.

"No, no sedation."

"Have you considered a nursing home placement for her?"

I responded to that with honesty, after releasing a long sigh. "There've been times that I've found the thought entering my mind, but, I want to stick it out at home as long as I'm able to keep her with those she knows, with family."

All of their questions were sparked by an alternate agenda. I'd heard them before. All were questions masking personal opinions that I'd heard time and time again. They were either voiced outright or cloaked in insinuations by medical professionals since Mary and I had begun the odyssey. No one seemed to get it, though. No one seemed to get why we voluntarily placed ourselves in the position of having to deal with someone with combative dementia on a twenty-four-hour basis.

Speaking from experience, it seems that, on the whole, society's simple solution—its pat answer—to my mother's condition is placement in a nursing home. Period. When Mom still had all her mental faculties and was as lucid as you and I, going into a nursing home was never considered as being a viable option for her own future. One of her greatest verbalized fears during the later stages of her life was contracting some type of dementia and, consequently, being faced with the possibility of ending up in a nursing facility. Well, although the first part of her fear did materialize, the second portion of it didn't. Although the dementia was unavoidable, a nursing home *was* avoidable. At least as long as this daughter was still around and continued to care about seeing that her mother's greatest fear was never realized.

Now, I would be less than honest if I didn't admit that Mary and I had considered a nursing home placement because, in such a complicated situation, with a patient's dementia condition growing worse by the day and the related aggressive behavior increasing, *all* options were considered and thoroughly discussed. All options. We'd agreed that Mary Belle would be cared for in a loving home until the end. We were both committed to that mutual decision.

Here we were, on the cusp of the new millennium, a society pregnant with technological advances, most of which had appeared in the last twenty-five years, and, in that same twenty-five years, we had created these "nursing homes" as a socially acceptable depository for our "problem" elders.

I'd personally thought a great deal about what families generally did before the advent of nursing homes. Look back into your family histories, when Grandma and Grandpa lived with their children when they could no longer live alone. For one thing, we didn't used to live as long as we do now. Life expectancy wasn't as great. Case in point, the doctors at the hospital told me that, if I hadn't given Mom that nitroglycerin pill when I did and called the ambulance, she would have been gone within an hour.

We're living longer with the help of medical technology. What has been so disturbing to me is that our moral wisdom has not kept pace. Our deference to spiritual ethics has waned in relation to keeping pace with our seemingly advancing technology. I looked at this elderly, frail woman who spent a good eighteen years of her own life feeding, clothing, and caring for my needs when I was young and who now needed similar care herself. So, when the medical professionals were so quick to ask me if I'd considered nursing home placement, my answer was, "She is my Mother."

Associated with this response, I've been asked about my own profession, having to trade my personal and professional goals for the job of being a full-time caregiver, having to literally put my life on hold. Yet I could find no greater profession than caring for another human being—blood relative or not. If this was the job I'd been given to do at that point in my life, then it was the job I must strive to do with an open heart. My friend Mary frequently receives correspondence from her readers who are mothers, writing to express how they feel as though they aren't free to find their "purpose in life" because family obligations are holding them back. I see our prime spiritual purpose as being one in which we care for one another the best we possibly can. Obligations and responsibilities to another are the spiritual priority.

There are many, many issues that desperately need to be explored concerning advancing technology and declining moral ethics—the increasing apathy of morality and human ethics. How is it moral to use technology to extend a human life when, in turn, no "quality of life" is offered for that extended life? Are you really ready for your children to admit you to a nursing home, or are you expecting to spend Christmas around the family tree?

One of these major issues is that of the medical industry's perspective regarding home care and finances. You see, the at-home caregivers receive no monetary assistance for their patient care from any government or insurance agencies. If my mother had been in a nursing home, the state would have picked up the complete bill for her full care. Why aren't those same funds available for in-home care? The way the societal cards are dealt, it would have been far more financially advantageous for us to place Mom in the nursing home. Her medical bills would have been covered and I could have once again worked outside the home. Yet, the cards are stacked against the home caregiver right from the start, because we alone bear the financial burden of having to carry the many additional expenses involved in having such a patient living in their home, such as paying for professional respite caregivers while you're away from the home attending to errands or appointments, or the expense of having to replace carpeting due to the patient's incontinence, or spending personal funds on sick room equipment, or having to replace furniture due to the patient's destructive behavior. At this point in time, government medical funding is only available to certified institutions or "certified" caregivers. Family members who bear the burden of such a loved one's care by helping to relieve the overcrowding nursing home situation are not included under this blanket of funding.

Mary Belle spent almost a week in the hospital, which is more than fifty miles from our home. I spent every day and long into the evening hours at her bedside and, every day, asked the doctors if I could bring her home. I repeatedly asked this, because the doctors themselves openly agreed that she was indeed stable enough to return home, and one physician actually had the audacity to admit to my face that the reason he wasn't willing to release her just yet was because, "If you needed to bring Mary Belle back in three or four days, the State Licensing Board would not look favorably at my decision to release her." So, ultimately, his decision to hold her in the hospital longer appeared to be based solely on state regulations and how his personal record would look rather than on a patient's wishes and welfare. And people ask why we don't have hospice workers come into our home to help? Same reason. Every medical professional wants to cover its legal backside by suggesting the service of the local hospice.

We had gone into the hospital with a new medical condition that needed to be stabilized and additional medications prescribed for it. Finally, after my mother was admitted on Sunday evening, we were able to take her home Friday morning. Because the doctors had been so indecisive, the nurses had left a Foley catheter in my mother the entire time. Yet she was entirely able to walk herself into the bathroom and use it unassisted. It was more convenient for them to keep her confined to the bed. I do not believe it was in her best interest or care. That Foley should have been out at least twenty-four hours before she was released. There were so many issues and details that you got lost in them.

The diuretics they were giving Mom depleted her potassium which, in turn, caused severe leg cramping. She had had this problem in the past and quinine sulfate tablets immediately relieved the pain. It took five hours for the hospital staff to get her this simple medication that I had at home in the medication cabinet. The frustrations were endless.

Eventually, on Friday morning the doctor signed the discharge papers. That morning, the doctors talked to me. They didn't focus their instructions on her medical care, but rather more on making sure it was on record that they discussed the advisability of getting hospice in to help with my mother's dying.

When I arrived home with Mom, Mary immediately informed me that both my brother and sister had called to tell us that they were on their way to Colorado. Somehow, they both decided that they needed to come out and were already en route. My reaction was mixed. It was mixed because I knew everyone would be glad to see each other, yet, on the other hand, Mother also really needed complete bed rest and emotional quiet to rebuild her strength. Flexibility is a must when dealing with people and their individual emotions. It's always a compromise to strive for that balance. Not only was Mother tired, I was too. Making the trip back and forth from the hospital was exhausting, and I wasn't quite prepared for housing and feeding company. All I wanted to do now was to get some much-needed rest. However, family was on the way. I understood their emotional need to be here.

Judy stayed two days, and Tony stayed through the week to help Mary and me get some cordwood cut, as that all-important fall project had been interrupted by the hospital stay. By spending an entire week with us, Tony was finally able to witness firsthand some of what Mary and I had been trying to describe over the phone about his mother's behavior.

I've noticed a funny thing about human nature through all of this. Folks will ask how things are going, but if you tell them the reality of it, their body language shows that they're sorry they asked and they will completely avoid asking the question when you next meet them. They also seem to think that you're somehow exaggerating the situation. No. No exaggerations. In fact, I actually toned down the behavioral incidents when I relayed them to folks. I didn't tell everything as I felt that that would somehow infringe on my mother's privacy. The way people don't want to hear bad things, and the extent they go to in order to avoid hearing them, leave me to wonder often just how long society can continue avoiding such world realities as the truth about the clinical behavioral symptoms of a disease like Alzheimer's.

While Judy and Tony were still here, Mary Belle had a second heart attack on the Sunday following her hospital discharge the previous Friday. During the second event, we remained at home, used the medications available, and she got through it. Overall she looked much more frail and physically tired. Her confusion and dementia had taken a drastic turn for the worse. Hallucinations were nearly constant, and she got anxious and agitated much more often and easily. Combativeness was a first reaction, then. An "attack mode" had become a first response behavior.

A week after my mother's second heart attack, I'd been out on errands and, upon returning home, found Mary desperately trying to assist an extremely combative Mary Belle up the stairs and into her room. Mary had just finished getting Mary Belle back from the woods—twice! She'd snuck out the first time when Mary was on the phone with a business call; and the second time my mother decided to take off up the drive was when Mary was in the basement starting a load of laundry. I found Mary in a nearly exhausted state from twice retrieving my combative mother from the woods and then trying to get her to go up to the safety of her room. Mary is a small-boned woman, not weighing more than 110 pounds, and not much stronger than my mother when she got into one of her aggressively combative states.

When I arrived, Mary Belle had been holding on to the cedar stair post with a death grip, refusing to budge up the stairs, all the time cussing at Mary and trying to bite her hands. I dropped my packages and rushed over to help. Even with my added assistance, it was rough going, because Mary Belle purposely slumped into a dead weight and refused to expend any effort into helping us get her up the stairs. By the time we'd managed the feat by carrying her up, we were both huffing and puffing with pounding hearts. Once in her room, Mary Belle settled down and promptly forgot the entire incident. When reminded, she claimed that we were making it all up . . . telling lies again.

The very next morning, Mary and I were sitting in the living room in our robes with our first wake-up cup of coffee. Mary Belle, all dressed and chipper, came down the stairs with her dog. We heard her let Molly outside and waited for her to join us. She didn't. The next thing we heard was the Nova's engine starting up.

In our bare feet, we rushed out the door (our drive is comprised of dirt and sharp pieces of natural, Rocky Mountain granite gravel). I reached the car just as my mother shoved the gear into reverse. Once I got her out, she flashed me a hateful look and decided she was going for a leisurely stroll up the drive. We let her go, figuring that she'd tire quickly and come right back down. Mary and I returned to the living room where Mary kept an eye on Mary Belle through her chair-side window.

The next thing I know, Mary is looking out that window and exclaiming, "Oh God, Mary Belle's climbing into the Jeep!" The Jeep is an old one with a plow on it. I'd left it parked up at the turnaround with the keys in the ignition after grading the drive the previous day.

Again I rushed outside, scrambled into the pickup, and pulled it up behind the Jeep's bumper so that Mary Belle couldn't go anywhere. When I went over to the Jeep and opened the door, I told Mary Belle to get out and come back down to the house.

She muttered, "Let's see, where'd I put that thing?" Then she found what she was looking for—her weapon. She picked up the long-handled ice scraper and began trying to hit me in the face with it. "I'm gonna *kill* you!" she kept screaming.

I managed to dodge her attempted blows and make purchase on her striking arm. She quickly twisted it out of my grasp. Her thin skin bruised. "Look what you've done to me! You *bruised* me! Ohhh, look! It's *bleeding* now!" And it was bleeding. Her thin skin would bruise and bleed at the slightest injury, which is why we tried to keep her in long-sleeved shirts, so that the little dogs jumping up on her would not cause injury to her wrists and arms.

I talked my mother out of the Jeep while she was concentrating on her wound. I talked her out by telling her that we needed to get back to the cabin to take care of her "wound." I drove us back down to the house and got her inside, where she then proceeded to kick me in the shin. When I turned to face her, she began hitting me with her fists. Mary came over to help, and we guided Mother to her chair. After bandaging her arm, we all sat down to catch our breaths.

Mary Belle appeared to calm down.

That was wishful thinking.

Suddenly she shot up out of her chair, strode with purpose across the room, and began pummeling me about the head and shoulders with her fists again.

I stood and tried to grab her arms. Mary came up and took one arm while I held the other, and we guided my mother toward the stairs. We had to get her back into her room, where we could distract her thoughts and get her mind occupied with something other than her obvious intent on doing physical harm to one of us.

Again she grabbed the cedar stair post with that death grip, and we had to pry her fingers off of it. Once we got her centered between us, Mary Belle decided to slump into her dead weight position, refusing to be of any assistance in getting her upstairs (acting much like protesters at a demonstration rally who slump in limpness when the police attempt to pick them up). We had to literally support her entire body and inch her up the stairs one at a time while she dragged her legs behind her, kicking her feet, and biting at our hands.

We managed to get her into her room and sitting in her chair, but she immediately shot up out of it and began to frantically search the room for something to wield as a weapon. "I'm going to *kill* you!" she screamed over and over again. I locked the door and found Mary hunched over, sitting on the top step, puffing hard with the effort to catch her breath. Don't forget, we're at an elevation of nearly 10,000 feet here and that kind of physical exertion can start the heart pumping hard— really hard. The rest of the day was near normal and there were no more incidents.

At 6 the following morning, we were awakened by screaming. Mary Belle had opened her bedroom dormer window and was bellowing at the top of her lungs. "*Help*! *Help*! They're KILLING me! They're *killing* me!"

We raced into her room, and she immediately began kicking out at both of us. We managed to get her seated in her recliner before rushing out the door and locking it behind us. As we heard her begin to scream out the window again, I raced downstairs to return with hammer and nails. When I again entered her room, my mother turned to me with fire in her eyes and fists raised. "I'm going to *kill* you! And *then* I'm getting out of here through that *window*!" I managed to safely maneuver around her flailing fists and nail the window shut while she was busy searching around for something to hit me with.

When I next returned to her room to bring her the morning heart and blood pressure medication, she threw the handful of pills onto the bed shouting, "Those will *kill* me! If I take those I'll be *dead* and *you'll* be the one who *killed* me!" (Again, this comes from the "preoccupation with death" symptom.)

I quickly gathered up the pills and handed them back to her. Utilizing her own fear of becoming constipated, I calmly said, "Mother, if you don't take these pills you'll get constipated." She immediately reached for them and swallowed every last one.

The following day was a fairly calm one, but when I went into her room to give her lunch, I was shocked to see that the dark pine finish on Mary's new hutch dresser top was deeply gouged out—in many places. I was mortified. "Mother!" I exclaimed, "What'd you do to Mary's furniture?"

"Nothing," came the highly defensive reply. "Why do you always think I do things? Why do you lie like that and make accusations?"

"I'm not lying. I ask things like that because that damage wasn't there this morning. And nobody else has been in this room but you. What'd you use to gouge out the wood like that?"

The conversation was a total waste of time because she kept denying having done it. Yet, later in the afternoon, while Mary was downstairs working at the computer, she heard scraping sounds coming from Mary Belle's room and went up to see what was causing it. Mary Belle was using a metal hair clip and a piece of sharp jewelry as carving tools to dig more finish off the dresser. "Mary Belle!" she shouted, catching my mother in the act. "What're you doing?"

"Ohhh, I'm just fixing this dresser," came the nonchalant reply.

Mary took away the makeshift carving tools, and I went through my mother's room in search of any and all sharp objects. When we later discovered her using her earrings and bracelets to do more creative carving on the bedroom set, I removed her jewelry box amid screams. "You're stealing all my things!" It did no good to spend time explaining to my mother that those "things" were being used as "tools" to destroy the furniture, because she'd just come back with, "I didn't *touch* that furniture. I don't know *who* did that! Why are you always accusing me of things?" What I would have given to have a video tape to play back for her to view. Yet even that would elicit a defensive escapism comment that went something like this, "Well! I certainly don't ever *remember* doing that," as if her lack of memory served as a defense against culpability. Ergo, what's the use of even going through all the bother of video recording her in the act?

Two days later, I came home from doing errands and found Mary cleaning the upstairs bathroom. Mary Belle had shoved her entire lunch down the bathroom sink drain and the toilet—both had overflowed when Mary Belle tried to wash it down and flush the toilet. Mary had just finished plunging out the clog and sopping up the floor and the soaked hallway carpeting.

Due to the latest idiosyncrasy of Mary Belle's, to dispose of her foodstuff down bathroom drains, we had to resort to the solution of confining her to her bedroom during mealtimes. That not only saved the plumbing and septic, but it also let us actually see just how much she was really consuming. Clearly, it taught us that we'd been mistaken to believe that she'd been eagerly finishing up all of her meals when, in fact, the meals had been going down the drain—literally.

And so we reached the "Retaliation" stage, where violence, thoughts of doing harm to others, and destructive behavior were the norm. Yet there was still balance. Oh yes, there was still some balance to be found.

One sunny autumn afternoon, we heard my mother having a lively conversation with many people in her room. We heard her easily because her room has an open wall, much like a loft area opening that looks down on the staircase. Of course, she couldn't get over it because it was blocked off with the heavy bedroom furniture, but sounds from her room traveled easily through the cabin.

So, on this beautiful, Indian summer day, we heard her having this very proper and cordial conversation. Hearing this from downstairs, Mary and I looked at one another, then silently crept up the stairs to peek over the ledge into her bedroom. We couldn't believe our eyes. When Mary looked back at me I could see hers were misting with welling emotion. We opened the locked stair gate at the top of the landing and entered the room.

All the room's chairs were lined up facing both sides of the bed. Stuffed animals were occupying every chair. Imaginary cookies and paper cups of water were at each place setting along the edges of the bedspread.

My mother was having a tea party.

When she saw us her eyes sparkled like Christmas tree lights. "Ohhh," she happily exclaimed, while clapping her hands like a small child filled with wonder. "Did you come for cookies and ice cream?"

We said that we had and graciously thanked her for inviting us.

It was the best tea party ever, more grand than an Inaugural dinner . . . love made it so.

A World Apart

The retaliation stage lasted approximately fourteen months. During that time Mary Belle exhibited her most physically aggressive behavior and corresponding verbal abuse toward us. After her second heart attack at home, her doctor advised us to try and keep her from climbing the stairs and wandering out of the cabin and up the drive. At such a high elevation, such activities were far too strenuous for such a fragile heart. Therefore, we made her bedroom as comfy as possible and even bought a sickroom toilet chair so that she wouldn't have to go as far as the bathroom to use the facility. We filled the room with all of her favorite, personal things and it ended up looking like a homey apartment. The gate at the top of the stairs remained locked at all times now, not just during the night. Mary Belle was at the stage where she understood that the stairs were indeed too much for her to handle and, on the whole, maintained an accepted attitude toward that situation. We brought her meals upstairs and she was content to eat them in front of her television or at her craft table with all of her stuffed animals placed in a semicircle around her plate.

However, the homey appearance of her little apartment only lasted for about three months. Throughout this retaliation phase of the disease, her once personalized bedroom became more bare and sterile than a hospital room. It was eventually devoid of all pieces of decorative items due to the fact that she perceived each piece of decor as being a potential weapon to wield, or as an implement of destruction. As caregivers, we felt some guilt over having to resort to creating such starkness in our loved one's world, but for Mary Belle's safety (and ours) we had no choice in the matter.

The many family pictures that were scattered about the room had to be taken away, as she'd remove the photos from the frames and use the sharp-edged glass to gouge the furniture and, ultimately, end up cutting herself. The ceramic Catholic statuettes were likewise removed because she would frequently become upset over something happening on her television and try to smash the screen with one of the figurines. We'd found puzzle pieces floating in the toilet water so the puzzles left the room. Her jewelry boxes went after she used them to scratch the furniture and to jab at us whenever she felt it necessary. The silk flower arrangements were taken away after she stood at the top of the stairs and threw them down over the gate in an attempt to hit the Yorkies with them. Even her favored small bed table lamps were removed after one broke as it hit the wall after she swung it at Sally. Eventually, there was nothing left in her room but the basic necessary furniture and her television. Tony sent her a collection of stuffed animals after we'd discussed their innocuous presence. Mary Belle perceived these as her "children" and could be heard disciplining them throughout the day.

Although the room was stripped, Mary Belle could still manage to find a weapon. One day, she didn't want to eat when Sally delivered a full dinner plate to her room, and she pulled out a small, empty dresser drawer and swung it at Sally. Luckily, my friend's reaction time was swifter than Mary Belle's swing.

Another time, when Sally brought her mother her morning pills and fresh coffee, Mary Belle threw the pills down the stairs and then tossed the hot coffee in Sally's face. Even a cup of coffee is perceived as a useful weapon during the retaliation stage. When the coffee was gone, the cup itself was used to hit Sally on the side of the head. When no weapons were within easy reach, the fingernails and teeth served just as well. I have a scar on my shoulder from being bitten when trying to help her remove her shoes for the night. And, she wouldn't hesitate to kick whenever it best suited her needs.

As I stated, the violent stage lasted for about fourteen months before a marked change occurred. Almost overnight, Mary Belle became much more docile. It was as though she no longer had the strength or inner resolve to expend energy on physical aggression. There were still times when she'd try to bite, dig her nails into our skin, and kick out with her feet, but those attempts were becoming less and less frequent.

This new phase in her behavior was like a semi-autistic one, because she was no longer able to comprehend sentences spoken to her. She could not come up with a related answer when asked a question. Her "conversations" with imaginary people increased, and she'd talk for hours in a nonsensical manner.

Mary Belle was now in her own little world apart from ours. Her reality was one completely different from that of society's. Most of the time she didn't know where she was or who either of us were. When her relatives phoned to speak with her—even her children, Tony and Judy—she wouldn't know who they were and would mentally drift into a one-sided conversation with herself, or, she'd simply set the receiver down on the bed and walk away, while leaving the other person hanging on the line.

On the whole, Mary Belle acted as though she didn't know who Sally was, yet we believe that familial bonds were extremely strong. We believe that Mary Belle somehow knew that she was living with family because, once in a blue moon, she'd shock us by calling Sally by her name. A couple of times she even called me Mary.

So although this "disconnected" late stage
would appear to mostly consist of behavior c[...]
associated from reality, we witnessed sparks of
nition that seemed to break through that i[...]
separating her world from ours.

Examples

Up until that point in time, the television had been a
wonderful diversion for Mary Belle. She'd sit in her recliner
and watch it for hours. Yet, now she'd lost the comprehension that the television was not always a true representation
of reality. She couldn't differentiate between the reality of a
newscast program and the make-believe of a soap opera or
movie. If there was some type of villain on the TV, she'd go
up to the screen and bang on it, "You no good, so-and-so.
I'm gonna kill you!" At this point, either Sally or I would go
upstairs and simply change the channel to a more innocuous type of programming. Mary Belle wouldn't even notice
that the change had been made and would sit back down
and again be drawn into the action on the screen.

More often than not, though, the television was something to be ignored. As time passed, she would seem to take
no heed that it was even on. Her past enjoyment taken from
watching it had appeared to wane considerably. Instead of
talking to the people on the screen, we'd hear her having a
lively conversation, and, when one of us went up to check
who she was talking to, she'd have her chair over in front of
the closet, talking to the hanging clothing. Other times
she'd be conversing with the bedpost. Many times the one-
sided discussion would be with her collection of stuffed animals. Although the interest in the television had diminished
to nearly nil, we still put it on in the morning for her and
didn't shut it off until bedtime.

There was no longer any sign of verbal comprehension
when we attempted to engage Mary Belle in a conversation.

quently, one of us would go into her room and sit on her bed to spend time with her. She seemed to prefer non-communication rather than being drawn into even the simplest of conversations. We'd like to think that she enjoyed the company, yet would react to such company in a disassociative manner of behavior. She'd forget you were there and talk to the stuffed animals or the television.

When Judy came out to Colorado and stayed a couple of days, she spent most of the time up in her mother's room. Not being able to draw Mary Belle into any logical conversation, she offered her opinion. "I think Mom needs more human contact."

No clue. Absolutely no clue in understanding the extent of Mary Belle's declining mental state. We could spend our entire day with Mary Belle in her room and it'd be as though we weren't even there. We knew this from experience. Being the sole caregivers, we'd taken extra steps to insure that our loved one had plenty of human contact. We were not solely her food delivery people or the maids who only entered the room to vacuum and change the bed. We had spent hours out of our day sitting with her and keeping her company. Yet, evidence of her acknowledging our physical presence was not there. More the contrary, it would always seem as though we were made to feel that we were actually unwelcome in her private domain . . . a presence to be barely tolerated.

Since the enjoyment of the television had waned to almost nothing, Mary Belle would occupy her time with other activities. One in particular was that of stripping her bed down to the mattress . . . three times a day. She'd take off the spread, the blanket, both sheets, the waterproof mattress cover we had to buy, and even the pillowcases. These would be placed in piles about the room, stuffed in desk drawers, or shoved into her toilet chair . . . after she'd used it.

When she initially began taking her bed apart, I'd go in and remake it for her. She'd sit in her recliner and tell me that I was doing it all wrong and attempt to push me aside so she could do it "proper." Yet she couldn't and would only end up becoming increasingly frustrated, soon working herself up into a state of high agitation. Her blanket was an electric one that Tony had bought her as a gift for Christmas. Since we heat the cabin with a woodstove only, Mary Belle would sometimes complain of being chilly during the long winter nights. Yet, in actuality, the heat from the living room woodstove rose directly up the stairs and into the stairway opening of her bedroom. She only "believed" that she was chilly when she saw the snow blanketing the valley below her dormer window. Many of her beliefs were generated by visual associations rather than actuality. When Mary Belle began her activity of stripping the bed, the blanket's connection cord would be pulled out of the bottom of the blanket and tightly wound around the bedpost. The plug would be pulled from the wall. It wasn't safe for her to be tampering with cords and electrical outlets so, like a parent who has to give attention to child-proofing the house, we disconnected the cord from her blanket and put it in the basement. Mary Belle never noticed that she no longer had artificial heat in her blanket. After we added a second quilt, she never again said she was "chilly" at night.

Yet I wasn't going to make up her stripped bed three times a day either. A caregiver quickly learns what is futile work and what is necessary to attend to. So if Mary Belle wanted to completely strip her bed down to the bare mattress in the morning, it stayed that way until bedtime. That way we only had to make it up once a day. While the bedding was off she'd occupy her time folding, unfolding, and refolding the sheets and blankets. She seemed to enjoy the activity. Perhaps it made her feel productive. There were times when she couldn't accomplish the feat of making a folded blanket; other times she appeared to delight in folding them and then moving them about the room, while deciding exactly where they should go until bedtime. It was interesting when the pillowcases frequently ended up being snuggle-type beds for her stuffed animals—as though she were putting her children into a nicely tucked-in bed. Then she'd carry them around that way and end up rocking them to sleep.

Another activity she'd engage in would be to take all of her dresser, nightstand, and desk drawers out and stack them on the bed. This ended up causing all manner of frustration when she attempted to put them back where they belonged. It turned out to be like a complex puzzle that she couldn't manage to piece together. She'd try for hours in an attempt to fit a dresser drawer into one of the desk openings. If you tried to assist her, she'd push you away, not wanting you to "touch her things." You wanted to help her out because you could see the incredible frustration she was putting herself through. You tried all kinds of reasoning, yet none of them were accepted. So you were left with the only alternative— you left her to do what she wanted to do. And that was to do it herself. And, of course, there were those days when she insisted that "on the *bed* is where the drawers *belong*." In that case, you didn't even try to help her put them away.

Rhymes. This end stage symptom of being in a world apart from reality was full of rhymes. She automatically interpreted the spoken word in rhymes. This was something we hadn't witnessed until she reached that stage. We're not sure if it was due to an inability to hear as well as she did before, or whether it was generated from some type of mental disassociation when hearing the spoken word. At any rate, the behavior had become routine.

After Mary Belle had finished a meal and I went into her room to collect her dinnerware (had to make sure the sharp forks and knives came back out), I'd look about the room. The plate and eating utensils wouldn't be on her table. They wouldn't be anywhere in sight.

"Mary Belle? Where's your plate?"

"Oh, really?" she'd reply.

"Where's your *plate*?" I repeat.

"Ohhh, I hate that too."

"Not *hate*, Mary Belle. *Plate*. Where . . . is . . . your . . . *plate*?"

She'd look around the floor. "Mate to the sock?"

It was at that point I didn't continue the conversation and went about searching the room for the missing plate and eating utensils. They might have been on the bookcase. They might have been in the her laundry hamper or in the toilet chair; her pockets or a pillowcase were common hiding places.

The first time she stripped her bed I asked her, "Why'd you strip your bed?"

She responded with, "No, I haven't *read* anything."

I pointed to the bare bed. "Your *bed*, Mary Belle. The bed. Why'd you strip it?"

"You tripped?"

More and more, it became the norm to experience nonsensical conversations. More and more, you learned that it was wise to save time (and frustration) by not even asking her questions that she had an inability to answer in a related manner. Yet that caregiver solution takes conditioning because when you walk into her room to bring her a meal and say something cheery like, "Come an' get it while it's hot!" She may respond with, "You got a rock? No, thanks."

Then, you'd naturally have an automatic reaction directed at trying to straighten out her misconception. "No, Mary Belle, your meal. Your *meal's* hot."

"A hot deal?" she exclaimed. "I'll say, what a deal that is."

Around and around went the verbal merry-go-round. So you ended up pointing to the steaming plate on her table, going over to her recliner, and helping her up and over to the waiting dinner. Even when she was in front of the table, she might not compute that her meal was set and waiting for her, because she might have said, "How can I eat if you don't bring it to me?" Then you had to put the fork in her hand

and place it to the plate. "Here, Mary Belle, see? Here's your food. It's all ready for you to eat."

"No, I don't need heat in here. I'm too hot."

At this point you didn't begin another round of nonsense by trying to explain that the reason she was too hot was because she had seven shirts on. At that point you left her with her meal and exited the room until she'd finished.

The appearance of the rhyming syndrome had the potential to deepen the caregiver's frustration if one let it. Oftentimes, turning it into a humorous situation alleviated that possible sense of futility and shifted it to amusement instead.

A world apart. A solitary world that exists within one's own mind. A world separate from the reality of others. This is an *end-stage behavioral phase* of the disease. The days when Mary Belle was off in this private world began to become the norm, rather than the exception, toward the end.

During this phase, she became fixated on her father. Everyone was "daddy." And there were days on end when she'd bang on her walls, calling and crying for him. She would moan and sob. "Daddy. Daddy. Daddy? Ohhh, daddy. please." Bang, bang, bang. "Please, daddy. Ohhh, daaaddy, please!" Bang. Bang. All day long we'd listen to this, and nothing we tried in an effort to break the sobbing cycle was successful. Once the "daddy" phase began, it continued on a daily basis until the end.

Along with this "daddy" period came other related behavior associated with her obvious immersion deep into her own world. There were many days when she'd be crawling around the bedroom floor on all fours making animal sounds. She'd bark like a dog or make gorilla noises. These were interspersed with hysterical laughter and bouts of the wracking-type sobs of real crying over imaginary situations that only she could see.

Frequently during this phase her mood would be dark and ugly. She'd exhibit a mean streak without any kind of provocation. She could even wake up in the mood. She'd laugh wildly and shout, "That man is gonna come an' *kill* you girls. *Then* you'll get yours!" Bang, bang on the wall. "Ha-ha! Then you'll get yours! Ha-ha-haaaa!" Bang, bang, bang, bang . . .

It was during this phase of the disease when our home began to continually sound more like the halls of Bedlam or Bellevue than a quiet and serene mountain cabin. The banging, pounding, hysterical laughter, crying, and shouting went on for hours at a time. There appeared to be no cognitive recognition of the patient's whereabouts, and we seriously wondered if this wasn't the time to place Mary Belle into a facility. Yet, to our amazement, she'd pull a complete surprise on us by hugging us and calling us by our right names. "Ohh, I love you, Sally," she'd cry. This, naturally, would throw us for a loop. Did it show that there were still moments of lucidity sparking from some shadowy corner of her brain, or was it merely pure chance that she'd managed to pull the correct name out of her memory base? It was a rarity when she called Sally "Sally" or me "Mary." And when she did, it caused us to think that perhaps there were still those exceptional times when she did know where she was and who we were.

Listlessness. The days between those spent banging on the walls all day, or laughing hysterically, or crying for her daddy, were frequently spent in an autistic-like listlessness when she'd do nothing but sit immobile in her chair and stare at the floor or wall. She couldn't be coaxed to eat or be cajoled into an interest in anything on the television. Efforts to engage her in any sort of conversation were unsuccessful. Her interest (or awareness) in anything was nil. It was much like watching the classic behavior of someone who was in the throes of a deep tunnel of severe depression. We'd try bringing a few of our dogs into her room to spark some kind of interest, because she always loved having the animals around her. Yet there would be no recognition of the pups' exuberant presence. It was like seeing someone sitting up in a coma with their eyes wide open but no possibility of physically or mentally stimulated interaction or recognition of the outside world.

Hygiene. This end-stage phase brought a marked decline in Mary Belle's attention to or recognition of personal hygiene. Though we'd placed a toilet chair in her room, she most often had no cognizant association of it being a place to use for elimination. Sometimes she'd urinate in it and then stuff her clothing into the removable bucket and close the lid. Other times she'd strip her bed and shove her bed sheet over her voided waste. However, most often she'd simply urinate wherever she pleased on the bedroom carpet—sometimes as much as three times a day. Frequently we'd find a pile of feces in the corner of her room. Once I found some in her sheets and had to search around the room for the main source that she'd taken it from.

Days that she'd defecate in her clothing and sit in it while watching her television were not uncommon. Her behavior appeared to be much like a baby's, who paid no mind to having to sit in soiled diapers. We'd have to argue and argue in an effort to convince her that she needed a shower and then she'd be physically combative with us the entire time. She wouldn't know what the soap was for. She'd wash behind her ears when told to wash between her legs. There was no understanding in response to the simplest instructions. Therefore, she'd bite and kick at us when we were forced to wash her ourselves in order to get her clean.

One day, when Sally was at work (she took a part-time job to help boost our declining income), I heard Mary Belle exclaim, "Ohh, it stinks! Ohhh!" I ran upstairs to find her slacks and the carpet full of diarrhea.

I eased her into the bathroom while she was trying to fight me. Getting her slacks and underwear down was a feat because she refused to lift up her feet so I could remove them. I tickled the bottom of her foot and she raised it enough for me to get one foot out of the clothing, then she stomped the foot smack down into the pile in the crotch of the underwear. Again I told her to raise her foot so I could help her get clean. She stepped off the clothing and onto the tile floor while, at the same time, reaching down to dig her nails into my neck. After managing to get her straight into the tub, I finished removing her soiled clothing. Her legs were coated with feces. I grabbed a towel to put the clothing in, while holding onto her to keep her from exiting the tub as she was attempting to do.

Just then Sally pulled up and, immediately hearing the commotion, raced up the stairs to take over the job. She was mortified that I'd had to take care of such a chore for her mother. Mary Belle fought with Sally the entire time her daughter worked to clean her up. She kept shouting, "You're killing me! Oh! Oh, you're killing me!"

Mary Belle had bathroom access all the time. However, Sally or I might have gotten up in the morning and stepped right into a fresh pool of urine on the hallway carpet. Sometimes Mary Belle wouldn't even bother to remove her clothing when she did it. She'd just stand in front of her television and urinate where she was standing, then not even realize that she was wearing soiled clothing. Keeping Mary Belle's bedroom clean and fresh had become on ongoing battle. The small Little Green Machine we were initially using wasn't getting it done any longer. We bought a major Hoover SteamVac to do a proper job of it.

One day when I was changing Mary Belle's bed and she was in the bathroom using the toilet, she'd kept the door opened and I passed by while going to the hallway linen cabinet for fresh sheets. What I saw her doing shocked me.

"Mary Belle," I exclaimed, "what're you doing with your hand? Get your hand out of there!"

"Gotta dig it out," came the reply.

I entered the bathroom and pulled her hand out from behind her. It was full of feces. She'd developed the habit of digging it out of herself.

Finally, our former mystery was solved. Lately we'd noticed that the right side of the toilet seat and sink faucet handles had feces smears on them once in a while and couldn't figure how it was happening. Well, there it was. Mary Belle had been using her hand to pull out her bowel movements, getting the feces on her fingers, using her hand to raise herself off the toilet, and then turning on the faucet to wash them. Good grief, what next? No wonder I was disinfecting the bathroom so much lately.

So during this phase of Mary Belle's disease, she considered it a necessity to "assist" in her defecation. It got to the point where one of us had to monitor every bathroom trip she remembered to make. If she defecated in her room we'd have to not only clean up the room, but put her into the shower or lead her to the sink to scrub her hands and fingernails good. If we missed an "event," we'd notice our omission when we'd see her sitting in her chair with a "dirty" finger in her mouth or up to her eye.

This decline in our patient's attention to elimination hygiene was a frustrating situation. We naturally tried putting diapers on her, yet she'd shred one piece by piece until she had it off and then hide the soiled pieces in her drawers or in between the sheets, sometimes even down in the pillow case. Putting the diaper on was always a physical battle because she didn't want to wear them and called us "mean" by making her wear them. Changing them was to take the chance of being bitten or scratched. Sally called several nursing homes to inquire how they handled patients who required diapers. They said that the patients wore a one-piece jumpsuit that zipped up the back to prevent them from being able to get to the sanitary underwear and tear it off.

We discussed this option and decided that it wasn't an option. Mary Belle was just too physically combative to allow us to peacefully undress her for the purpose of changing a soiled diaper. We concluded that the best course of action in our particular situation was to keep cleaning up the room, continue trying to monitor her every bathroom visit, and daily disinfecting all bathroom hardware including the door handle. Taking the risks of being bitten, kicked, and having fingernails dug into one's skin was not worth the effort to us. On the same hand, Mary Belle also risked injury to herself in these highly physical encounters that she instigated. If we left her alone, we would also avoid risking another heart attack brought on by her elevated blood pressure in fighting us over the wearing of clean underwear. Our choice made more work for us, but kept Mary Belle from becoming combative and prevented events that had the potential to greatly elevate her agitation level.

Mary Belle was at that stage when we took her out for a special treat. One September day, we drove her up to the top of our driveway where she and Sally got out of the car to take in the beauty of the mountain autumn afternoon. As they leisurely strolled down the drive, I followed in the car and, choosing certain places along the way, I took some photographs of mother and daughter enjoying the tranquil, fall day. We used one of these photographs for the cover of this book. Getting Mary Belle outside had become a rarity as she could no longer wear regular shoes due to her swollen feet. During this little excursion she was wearing a pair of Sally's sandals because none of her own shoes would fit her.

Upon our return to the cabin, Mary Belle squealed, "Ohh, look! Look at the lovely house! Who lives here?"

"You do, Mom," Sally smiled.

"I do?"

"Yes, you do. This is my and Mary's house. You live here with us."

"Well! That's the first I heard of that! Nobody told me that! Ohhh, this is sooo nice."

When we walked into the kitchen from the back door, she again exclaimed, "Ohhh, what a cozy place! Whose place is this?"

"It's mine, Mom," Sally repeated. "And you live here, too. This is your home."

"Oh."

Mary Belle was so exhausted from her little stroll down the drive that, once we helped her back up the stairs and got her settled in her room, she proceeded to make another puddle in the middle of her carpet before falling fast asleep in her recliner.

A week after the autumn photo shoot, I was awakened at 5:30 in the morning by a thump coming from Mary Belle's room. I ran across the hall and found her on the floor on her back, head bent up against the dresser. Blood was spattered on the carpet and beginning to already soak into the back of her shirt. She'd fallen. She'd fallen so hard against the dresser that the brass drawer pull was completely bent and torn from the wood.

I called for Sally and she came running. We got Mary Belle up off the floor. She was dizzy and weak. I supported her in an upright position in a chair while Sally went for a warm wash cloth to clean away the blood so that we could see what kind of injury we were dealing with. There was a three-inch gash in the back of Mary Belle's head and two hematomas were quickly rising from the base of her skull. We cleaned and wrapped the wound. Since we no longer had medical services of any kind in Cripple Creek and the nearest hospital emergency room was fifty miles away down in Colorado Springs, Sally drove her mother into Woodland Park, where Mary Belle's doctor had relocated.

Mary Belle was not the least bit cooperative. She was physically combative instead of helping the doctor help her. Sally had to hold both of her mother's wrists and wrap her other arm around Mary Belle's head to keep her still enough for the doctor to stitch up the wound. They left with instructions to watch for nausea or sleepiness.

When they arrived back home, I could tell that Sally had had one hell of a time by the look on her face. We got Mary Belle back up in her room and comfortably sitting in her recliner in front of the television. When I checked on her a half hour later, I discovered blood soaking into the back of her shirt—she'd been picking at the stitches. No amount of reasoning and cautioning would keep Mary Belle from fussing with her wound. She'd pull off any type of wrap we covered her head with. And all manner of contraption we devised to keep her hands away from the wound was not successful. Finally, we came up with one that kept the wound safe, yet frustrated our patient to no end because she couldn't get at the injury anymore. Heavy socks on the hands. And for the rest of the day and long into the night, we were bombarded by her nonstop ravings that we were "out to kill her."

As we sat down in the living room that evening trying to watch the summer Olympics in Sydney while blocking out Mary Belle's nonstop ranting, we both felt as though we'd reached wit's end and couldn't take another day of it. We are two individuals with exceptionally strong constitutions, yet, when a loved one reaches the behavioral end stages of Alzheimer's, those constitutions can be known to hang by a fragile thread. Eventually, our Mary Belle exhausted herself and, by well after midnight, we were finally able to fall asleep ourselves.

Another day dawned. It dawned with a brilliantly blue sky. An Indian summer day washed down over brightly colored leaves of shimmering gold and glistening amber. The sun was pleasingly warm and a light breeze shushed through the aspen leaves. The mountain air freshened the atmosphere and gave one the sense of breathing pure oxygen. The trees were full of ravens and crows. The valley was alive with birdsong. Squirrels were scampering along the pine branch porch rails. Life renewed itself with a brand new beginning. So did we.

Almost a week later it was Mary Belle's birthday. It didn't seem possible that another whole year had come and gone. Though she kept forgetting that it was her special day, she delighted in opening each brightly wrapped package and looking at the cards sent from friends and relatives. She attacked her box of candy like it was the first assortment of chocolates that she'd ever laid eyes on. Her head wound was healing nicely. And her overall health was maintaining itself. It was a good day. It was a day that shined like a sparkling diamond among the many gray stone days that surrounded it.

It was a good day.

It was duly recognized as such and counted as a blessing to be appreciated.

III. THE CAREGIVER'S TOOLS FOR SURVIVAL

Management through Basic Rationale

Remembering That Grain of Salt

This all-important caregiver tool is all about internalization. By this I'm specifically referencing that internalization frequently done by the caregiver that's directly associated with the *personalization* of the patient's behavior, and the use of wisdom to avoid being drawn into such a destructive, self-effacing emotional space. Simply put, don't take things personally. Never take things personally. This disease isn't about you. It's not about anyone other than the patient. And whatever types of mean-spirited words or statements are verbalized by the patient and are pointedly directed toward you as the caregiver, are not to be taken to heart and anguished over.

Alzheimer's is a disease of the brain. It seriously affects one's thought processes. When an afflicted loved one begins calling you all manner of names, you can't allow those names to become a spear in your heart and haunt your days. You can't torment yourself over the fact that your loved one no longer recognizes you, or agonize over the additional fact that the patient loses all compunction to strike out at you whenever the mood arises. Though these behaviors would appear to evince some kind of deep-seated hatred for the caregiver, that same aggressive behavior should never be internalized in a personal manner. The patient's behavior is being initiated by slowly degenerating brain cells, not by diminished love or parental bonds for the adult child who has taken on the job of her/his parent's care. These are two separate concepts which are imperative for the daily caregiver to always keep in mind.

Dealing with Alzheimer's is dealing with dementia. I repeat, *dealing with Alzheimer's is dealing with dementia.* Dementia. Though some so-called "experts" will claim that the disease is not the same as insanity, my own experience with it would tend to widely differ from that statement. I see that too-simple statement as being more of an opinion than one based on hard fact because pounding on walls all day long, crawling around on hands and knees barking like a dog, and rolling feces into marble-sized balls and hiding them around the room is not sane behavior. Hallucinating the bedpost as being her dog and trying to shove her dinner into its mouth, then become angry when it doesn't eat, is not sane behavior. Banging on her door for hours on end, while screaming that she wants to kill everyone she sees, is not sane behavior. And, if the routinely exhibited behavior isn't indicative of being sane, what is it? Is there some grey area between sane and insane? If so, was that where Mary Belle had journeyed to? So, I differ from those experts who would claim otherwise. And, it would appear that Sally and I are not the only ones to differ on this account, as we've spoken to many people who've been through the experience of caring for an Alzheimer's parent in their own homes, and they, too, have been quick to nod and agree that the end-stage phases are indeed nothing less than dealing with a situation of total insanity.

Some of these caregivers stuck it out to the end, others ended up placing their parents into a nursing facility during those completely irrational final stages, because they felt as though "one had to be mad to be able to deal with the madness twenty-four hours a day." To be honest, that same thought had crossed our own minds more than we'd like to admit, because there'd been days when we too thought we were going mad having to listen to someone banging on walls most of the day . . . and sometimes all night long. Or hearing someone instantly alternate from sobbing uncontrollably to laughing hysterically and, then, within a heartbeat, shift to making all manner of animal noises.

So, when the patient spews hateful names at you and says mean-spirited things, it's not the person who's talking, it's the disease. These shifts in mood can come on so swiftly that it can give the observer an eerie sensation, as though the patient had been suddenly possessed. This is not an exaggeration, as most experienced caregivers will quickly attest to experiencing this same skin-tingling sensation. The shift in altered mood and attitude can be accomplished with lightning speed. The afflicted loved one can be hugging you and, with tears of deep emotion flowing from her eyes say, "Oh, honey, I love you so. Thank you so much for putting up with me and taking care of me." And *blam*! The next minute, the arms that were so lovingly wrapped around you will rise, poised high in the air, before coming down in a hard blow to your head or back. Or, the hands that were gently stroking your back will suddenly spring talons and begin to dig in. The shift looks and feels very much like possession or multiple personality syndrome. Sane behavior?

For the caregiver to take these incidents of aggression, no matter how quickly the change in mood occurred, as being personal serves no constructive purpose for that caregiver. That type of psychological internalization only ends up causing the caregiver unnecessary grief and, therefore, has the potential of generating a host of exponential negative responses, such as resentment, toward the afflicted loved one.

When Mary Belle called one of us her favored, "Snot-Slut" name, we didn't take it personally. When she shouted in our faces, Liar! or Murderer!, we let those roll off our backs. It's the disease doing the name-calling, not the old

Mary Belle who would've been absolutely mortified to hear herself talk in such an unkind, socially unacceptable manner. When she flung the empty dresser drawer at Sally's head, my friend didn't take it personally because she knew that it was the disease causing the aggressive behavior. When I bent down to help Mary Belle remove her shoes for the night and she proceeded to bite my shoulder, I didn't take it personally. Sure it hurt. It drew blood and left a scar. Sure I immediately reacted with anger, but not at *her* . . . I reacted to the *behavior* that caused injury. That behavior is not personal. Although, on the surface, it would appear to be, it's not. It's definitely not. It's the result of an uncontrollable urge to strike out at anyone or anything who's within closest proximity to the patient at the time. She'd strike the bedpost if it was closest. This, of course, would leave a large bruise on her hand and then she'd accuse one of us of causing it. That wasn't personal either. It wasn't personal when she did it all by herself—to herself. So, why take verbal and physical aggression directed against yourself as being personal if the patient can direct it just as intently toward a bedpost?

Recognizing the fact that it's the disease that's behind the patient's aggressive behavior, and not the patient's formerly lucid mind, goes a long way in serving as a golden key for the caregiver to utilize. Taking everything with that little "grain of salt" helps to provide more effective patient care and, at the same time, insulates the caregiver's emotional sensitivities against unwarranted and unwanted feelings and attitudes. These can become self-defeating and destructive elements in the caregiver's life. These can often make the caregiver feel as though he/she isn't loved by the afflicted parent or, perhaps even more devastating in the long-term, bring on that commonly recognized "sense of false guilt" by germinating thoughts that something must be amiss with the quality of care being provided. These negative attitudes will seriously affect that quality of care one strives so hard to give. By taking everything the patient says and does with a grain of salt, these damaging attitudes can be avoided. Remember to never internalize the patient's behavior. By doing that, the caregiver avoids complicating the issue by compounding the situation with personal emotional clutter. Leave yourself out of it. Keep it simple!

It's not personal. It's the disease.

It's only the disease.

Out of Harm's Way

Safety. This tool is associated with maintaining the physical safety of the patient and also that of the caregiver. It's related to personal and environmental safety. Providing a safe home environment for your afflicted loved one is much the same as "child-proofing" a house as a preventative measure when the grandchildren come by. Except, in this case, the "child" is usually over five feet tall and can reach a multitude of potentially hazardous items, such as the knife block on the kitchen counter and the stovetop burner and oven knobs.

When the disease progresses to the later stages of mental deterioration, the caregiver realizes that the most innocuous household items and decor can become a threat to the patient's safety. Those family photographs hanging on the wall in the loved one's room can be taken down, dismantled, and the sharp framing glass used as a lethal weapon. That bedside boudoir lamp that had been in the patient's family for as long as anyone can remember may suddenly be perceived by the patient as a convenient club to wield. The simple spoon can be hidden away to later use as a jabbing device, and jewelry is loaded with pins and sharp edges. I once caught Mary Belle trying to chew on the beads of one of her necklaces, thinking they were candies.

We naturally felt twinges of guilt when we discovered that we had to remove most of Mary Belle's personal items from her room. One by one, as she used them for destructive purposes, items came out and went into storage boxes. Week by week, as her behavior worsened, the room became more sparse. Yet what was interesting was that she never noticed that items were disappearing from her room. She never missed one of them. She never searched around for anything that had been removed. It was as though those things never existed, so thoroughly were they forgotten. And so the initial guilt over having to remove so much from her room dissipated due to the realization of her apparent nonchalance over the entire issue.

Some of the Alzheimer's reference books we read made suggestions for dealing with this critical situation of safety. The solution was to hide all sharp kitchen utensils, remove the knobs from the cookstove, and empty drawers containing potentially hazardous items. To us, this was no solution at all because the microwave was still sitting there, as well as a multitude of other various potentially dangerous items such as the toaster, coffee maker, and eating utensils in the drawer. All were extremely hazardous to an Alzheimer's patient, as Mary Belle had poked a knife down in a glowing toaster, placed aluminum foil in the microwave, flipped on the coffeepot element switch when no liquid was in the pot, and hoarded forks in her pockets.

My point is that, for the twenty-four-hour, at-home caregiver, the home cannot be stripped and everything hidden away in the basement or placed under lock and key. That's just not reasonable because, eventually, *everything* in the home may be perceived as a potential weapon or harmful item to the patient. So when that patient reaches this stage of the disease, the caregiver does what the mother of a new toddler does—she removes the child from harm's way and places the youngster in a safe environment, usually a playpen or other such secure place. Neither mother nor caregiver can continually shadow the child or patient all day long for the purpose of insuring the other's safety. Therefore, this was the stage when it became necessary for Mary Belle to live in a secured environment, where her exposure to possible harm was kept at a minimum. Our solution was twofold. By restricting her downstairs access, we provided her with an "apartment-type" environment and also removed the physically strenuous hazard of having to manage the stairs throughout the day. This latter problem was a great concern for us after her doctor strongly recommended that she not use the stairs at all following her two heart attacks.

Yet, even after Mary Belle's environment consisted of her large bedroom and the upstairs bathroom, she still found dangerous items within them. We had to remove all manicure and shaving utensils from the bathroom drawers. Even something as innocent-appearing as the box of cotton swabs became a problem and had to be taken out of her sight. Combs with rat-tail handles were removed as well as anything nonedible (she once squeezed the contents of a tube of antibiotic ointment onto her toothbrush). The bathroom paper cups had to be taken out after she tried flushing them down the toilet. Same with giving her snacks on paper plates. We soon converted all her dinnerware to the ironstone type, due to her habit of attempting to dump and flush her meal—plate and all— into the toilet.

Though we patient-proofed the upstairs bathroom by removing most of the medical items and potentially dangerous objects, we could live with that. Those things were either put in my bedroom for our own easy access, or they were added to the downstairs bathroom supplies. This solution was a small inconvenience, compared to the greater alternative of taking the chance of our loved one doing herself harm.

Once Mary Belle had the run of the upstairs, we had to put a keyed lock on my bedroom door to keep her from going in and helping herself to whatever she wanted. Again, there was the potential for harm from my jewelry boxes, pens on my computer table, the incense lighter, etc. Also, I needed to protect the current stack of printed-out papers of the working manuscript from disappearing. She once poured an entire bottle of Opium perfume down the bathroom sink—the perfume I'd received as a Christmas gift. Did I mind having to use a key every time I wanted or needed to get into my bedroom during the day? Sometimes. Sometimes I did, especially when it was laundry day and it was necessary for me to make many trips up and down the stairs loaded down with hampers and lugging around freshly ironed clothing on hangers. But still, compared to the alternative, those moments of frustration were nothing but a drop in the bucket. Having Mary Belle safe upstairs was a great comfort to us, knowing that she wasn't getting into the kitchen utensil drawer, turning on the stove burners when our backs were turned, or getting into my manuscripts.

So once Mary Belle was safe in her little apartment, we automatically thought that the "safety" situation was resolved. . . until she began finding things in her room that proved hazardous to her—and us. Her religious statuettes became a knocker to bang on the television screen whenever she didn't like how someone was behaving "in there." Or the figurines were handy little items to throw down the stairs at us or the Yorkies whenever we passed by the stairway. These were one of the initial items to be removed from her room. She never missed them.

The jewelry in her various jewelry boxes became carving tools with which to gouge out the tops of the dark pine dressers and night tables. Or, as I mentioned earlier, she'd attempt to eat a string of pearls, thinking they were candy. The jewelry boxes went next. They were never missed because she'd gone far beyond any interest in wearing such adornments.

Writing utensils were then used for the same gouging purpose. Mary Belle couldn't write her own name anymore, so there was really no reason why she needed those types of items in the rolltop desk Sally had placed in her room at the outset. Also, she found that a sharp pencil made a wonderful knife with which to jab at us if she found reason or inclination. All sharp writing utensils vanished from our patient's sight and access.

We naturally never gave a thought to all of those framed family photographs that we'd hung on Mary Belle's bedroom walls to make her feel at home. Yet, when I went into her room one morning to change her bed, she'd had three of the large pictures completely dismantled and spread out like puzzle pieces on her bed quilt. She'd cut her hand on the sharp glass edges, then blamed me for causing her wound. So, these, too, disappeared. She never noticed they were no longer there. As a substitute, we placed some of her photo albums on her nightstand. Family was still kept close by and she spent hours looking through the photographs wondering "who all these people were." Her recognition of family members and old friends had waned to nearly nil. However, the progression of the disease had reached the point when it was no longer important to her if she recognized these people or not, because her mind interpreted these photographs in an alternative manner. She perceived them as living people who were physically visiting her apartment and she spent hours involved in deep conversation with them. Since there was little she could successfully do anymore to occupy her time (simple projects were too difficult and she could no longer read), talking to these "visitors" was a way of passing the day away. . . and sometimes, the night, too.

When Mary Belle pulled the dresser hutch top down on herself, that gave us one hell of a scare. The noise was terrible and while racing up to her room, we'd envisioned her on the floor and bleeding, perhaps lying with a broken bone or two. The worst case scenario was not manifested and she'd come out of the mishap luckily unscathed. The dresser hutch also was removed. Little did we ever envision or imagine that she'd do such a thing, much less be physically capable of tipping over such a massive piece of heavy pine furniture on herself. Yet, for all of her ninety-seven pounds, she did manage to do just that. Fortunately the top of the hutch caught the bedposts and created a space in which she'd been spared. We felt blessed that the mirror didn't shatter over her in a rain of sharp shards.

One of Mary Belle's favored pieces of furniture was brought out here by Sally and placed in her mother's bedroom. This was an antique bookcase that revolved on a swivel base. It held a considerable number of volumes. Some of these volumes were themselves collectibles—antique, padded leather covers over one hundred years old. When we found Mary Belle ripping pages out of these precious books and peeling the stiff leather off the covers, they were quickly rescued and taken down to the bookshelves in the living room. She no longer had any concept of their value as she sat busying herself like a small child ripping pages out of an old magazine. She didn't remember how long they'd been in the family, nor did she have a care toward their collectible worth in the marketplace. Also, because Sally had given up her bedroom for her mother, she had many of her own books on that revolving bookcase. After seeing what her mother had done with the antique volumes, Sally decided it would be best to remove those of her own that she considered special and irreplaceable. So the bookcase was duly thinned out. We left only those volumes that Mary Belle could look through and that could be destroyed without concern. We also added replacements for those that'd been removed. These were of the "picture book" variety that Mary Belle liked to spend hours perusing. They were books like travel guides, AAA Tour Books, and our *Colorado* and *Natural History* magazines. We filled up the empty bookcase spaces with the stacks of women's magazines that had amassed from the subscriptions Tony had gotten for his mother. Mary Belle was happy with the new arrangement. So were the remaining antique books that rested safely down in the living room.

Another favored item of Mary Belle's that was brought out to Colorado was a floor lamp that Sally put in her mother's room. That, too, she pulled down on herself, and that, too, was removed, because it had glass globes that could shatter. Again, we were lucky that they remained whole when they hit the floor.

One sunny autumn afternoon, when Sally was out on errands, I heard the water running in the upstairs bathroom sink. It ran and ran. I heard Mary Belle agitatedly disciplining a small child. "I've got to wash behind your ears! Hold still!"

Child? What child?

I raced upstairs. "What're you doing, Mary Belle?" I asked, while unlocking the stairway gate.

"Ohhh, just giving this little guy a bath."

Upon entering the bathroom, I saw the wooden schoolhouse clock in the sink . . . soaked. She'd taken it down from her bedroom wall and decided it needed a good washing behind the ears.

"Mary Belle, that's a clock."

"Lot you know," she grumbled. "He's gotten himself all dirty."

I knew from experience that logic would not resolve the situation. I went into her bedroom and returned with a stuffed animal. "Here," I offered, "this boy's nice and clean. He's really sleepy and needs to take a nap."

Her eyes brightened as she eagerly reached for the gorilla. She whispered to it. "See? I *told* you to take a nap now," she said while jabbing her finger in its stomach. "Now I'm going to put you to bed, and you better stay there or else!" Away she went with the little boy, completely forgetting about the other one who needed his ears washed.

Diversion. Most of the time it worked like a leprechaun's charm.

I quietly wiped the timepiece off and took it down into the basement. Even her clock was now gone from her bedroom wall. The whole room was getting very bare and sterile looking, yet the new environment was created by Mary Belle's own behavior. We would've liked nothing more than to have her room full of all those personal things that she once loved. However, the key word there is "once." She didn't love any of those things anymore because she couldn't remember ever possessing and cherishing them. Whether her room was packed with personal items or as sparse as a bear's cave made not a bit of difference to her. Therefore, our guilt over having to remove so much was assuaged by her obvious indifference. She was content with what was remaining. Even the television held little interest for her anymore. Though we always left it on, she'd sit facing the closet thinking the clothing on hangers was children she could talk to and discipline.

As primary caregivers, your job is to keep your loved one as physically safe as possible. If removing the dresser hutch with the mirror she loved to have conversations with means keeping her safe, then that's what you do. If taking the wall clock away and having all the framed family photographs vanish from her room insures that safety factor, then that's what needs to be done. Having your loved ones cut themselves on glass from a dismantled picture frame is not being a conscientious caregiver.

You can carefully scrutinize your loved one's living environment with a sharp eye to safety and be absolutely certain that there's not a thing remaining in it that will cause harm, yet eventually, the patients themselves will clearly point our your error in judgement. Even a pillowcase can turn to disaster.

One evening when I brought Mary Belle a snack a few hours after dinner, I found her sound asleep in her chair. She had both feet snugly tucked into a pillowcase. If she'd awakened and tried to stand and walk away, she would've promptly fallen, perhaps hitting her head on the bedpost. Without waking her, I eased the case off of her stocking feet and put a new one on her pillow. Out of sight, out of mind.

When I woke her for her snack, she didn't remember that she'd tucked her feet into the case.

Safety. For someone caring for a late-stage-Alzheimer's loved one, safety can be a tricky commodity to come by. Frequent observation of the patient's behavior can point the way toward potential hazards and avoid a future mishap.

A sparse room is not a neglectful room.

A sparse room is a safe room.

Mary Belle's sparse room was filled with magazines, stuffed animals, and photo albums that replaced the glass-framed family pictures. Mary Belle's room was exactly how she wanted it. She was happy in what she called her "little apartment."

Happy and safe.

What more could a caregiver and his/her loved one ask for?

Know Your Meds

As I previously recounted when detailing the incident I experienced with the reaction to Mary Belle's sleeping medication, it's important for the caregivers to thoroughly understand everything about the prescription medications they're dispensing to their patient. Do some research and familiarize yourself with the conditions each specific drug is most frequently prescribed for. Prescription drugs are usually accompanied by a detailed information sheet that lists cautions and warnings, contraindications, drug and food interactions, possible side effects, overdosage, and special information to be on the lookout for. These are important for the caregivers to become thoroughly familiarized with so they can watch the patient for any sign of an adverse reaction and know which foods will be incompatible with the drugs.

Through attentive observation, the caregivers need to note if the patient is perhaps getting too high a dosage or too little. Are there any physical or behavioral changes in the patient after a new drug is introduced? Every individual's physiology and drug tolerance are unique because chemical levels vary greatly from one individual to another. Each person's tolerance for drugs is different and, depending on a wide variety of their other existing conditions, a physician may have to experiment through a trial and error selection of various prescription options to discover which one is least problematical for the patient to tolerate. Sometimes it takes a while for a doctor to zero in on the one drug that will prove most compatible for her patient. As the primary caregiver, you may possibly be the best source of information for the doctor, as your Alzheimer's patient will not normally be able to remember or describe her/his reactions to different medications. Also, many of these medications have a half-life or a lingering residual effect for a few days after they've been discontinued. Stopping a specific medication will not automatically mean that its chemical elements aren't still present within the body.

A commonly recognized physiological symptom accompanying Alzheimer's is that of choking. Before Mary Belle came to live with us she'd occasionally had some trouble swallowing and would have an outpatient procedure done at a Kansas City hospital to correct the recurring condition. Shortly after she arrived in Colorado, she again began having difficulty swallowing. Sally scheduled her mother with a Colorado Springs hospital to have a repeat of the "throat-stretching" procedure called an *esophageal dilation*. Although the operation was performed as requested, the specialist determined that Mary Belle's esophageal dysfunction was due more to a failing ability of the esophagus to maintain normal rhythmic contractions.

Whenever we eat anything, the esophagus contracts in a sequentially rippling motion along its length in order to effectively move foodstuff downward through it and into the stomach. Mary Belle's esophagus no longer contracted in a smooth, consecutive motion from top to bottom; rather it did so in a random manner. Her esophageal contractions were haphazardly occurring along its length between the throat and stomach, causing her to feel as though she were choking when making attempts to swallow food. The food was essentially hanging up on the *random* contractions instead of being naturally propelled downward in one smooth motion of consecutive contractions.

In this case, an esophageal dilation was not the ultimate answer. The answer, this particular physician determined, was a drug specifically designed to regulate those troublesome random contractions. This drug would re-regulate the natural order of the esophagus's consecutive contractions and, therefore, prevent further choking episodes. What one doctor missed, another caught. Not an unusual occurrence in our personal experience with the medical profession.

Thereafter, whenever we observed Mary Belle beginning to have some difficulty eating because she'd have some trouble swallowing, we immediately advised her to stop eating and take one small pill. After she waited five or ten minutes, giving the chemical time to work, she could successfully continue eating without further problems. This was not a daily, routine medication. It was only given upon evidence of difficulty swallowing. It would effectively work within minutes of ingestion.

The name of this drug was Propulsid. After we'd been intermittently giving it to Mary Belle for over a year and a half, we watched a television news broadcast disclosing the possibility of Propulsid causing heart attacks in patients taking it—even in children. We received no official advisement call from the doctor who'd originally prescribed the drug for his patient. We received no warning letter associated with the chemical from the physician's office. We didn't have to. Immediately we withdrew the drug from our medicine chest and no longer dispensed it to Mary Belle.

Needless to say, due to Mary Belle's chronic heart condition, we were greatly disappointed that this drug was proving to cause some fatalities in those taking it. We were even more disappointed that no new individual warning regarding its continued use was issued from the specific medical source that prescribed it to patients. If we hadn't heard of the research discovery broadcast on the television news program, we would have continued to give Mary Belle medicine that possibly could have done her more harm than good. Thankfully, we also discovered that, upon cessation of the drug ingestion, she seemed to no longer need it. Her choking problem rarely recurred. The incidents of choking had subsided, and we had no need to resort to an alternate drug. We were grateful that we didn't have to add yet another prescription to her round of medications. On the few occasions when Mary Belle seemed to begin having a bit of difficulty swallowing, we gave her a small Bayer aspirin. She believed it was her normal choking medication, and the mind did the rest as it prevailed over matter. The replacement pill, whenever needed thereafter, did the job as effectively as the former medication did. Eventually, Mary Belle's trouble with choking while eating disappeared altogether.

Because of the naturally occurring, clinical nature of the Alzheimer's disease and the manner in which the patient's brain cells progressively deteriorate, the brain's ability to continue insuring that the body's involuntary functions maintain normalcy also begins to noticeably wane and ultimately fail. The choking incidents are frequently a classic "onset" signal of this stage of deteriorating brain function, as they directly relate to the brain's former ability to keep the body working normally. Eventually, other involuntary body functions will follow suit. Instances of incontinence begin and accelerate in frequency. A recognizable lack of gross motor skills such as balance and generalized motor coordination is in evidence. Losing the simple hand-to-mouth ability to feed oneself, etc. begin to exhibit themselves as being intrusive elements that make their debilitating way into the patient's daily life.

Sally had become acutely sensitive to her mother's "health state signs," in that she could readily intuit if the blood pressure was too high and her mother needed an extra

Norvasc pill, or if she suddenly required absolute rest and an additional Nitrostat. I believe that this was a natural course for most familial caregivers—the natural development of a type of prescience associated with a loved one's current state of being. There appears to be a special connective bond that forms between the loved ones, almost like an umbilical cord.

Mary Belle never felt the inclination to advise us when she was experiencing a pain in her chest or when she thought her blood pressure had skyrocketed. Fortunately, we didn't need her to tell us these things because we could see what was happening by the way she looked or was behaving. This is a skill that becomes invaluable to the caregiver. It's a skill that carries the potential of being an eventual lifesaver, because I'd witnessed countless times when Sally had caught a certain expression on her mother's countenance or perceived a subtle nuance in Mary Belle's speech pattern or tone of voice that set the warning bells ringing for Sally to take corresponding countermeasures.

While I'm on the subject matter of medication, I feel the need to also include the importance of actually watching the patient take those medications. This is an essential tool we've learned to use through experience. Observance. The caregiver needs to *observe* the patient *ingest* the medication.

There were times when Mary Belle would attempt to fool us by pretending to take them. She'd "palm" them, hide them under her tongue until we turned our backs or walked away, or perhaps she'd surreptitiously "drop" some into her clothing or chair, or nonchalantly fuss with her hair and deposit the pills there. Also, even if the patient isn't into this particular type of chicanery, it's easy for them to mistakenly drop some of their pills, creating a dangerous situation whereby young children or inquisitive pets could accidentally ingest them.

During the paranoia stage of the disease, Mary Belle would adamantly (and often quite animatedly) claim that "the pills were positively going to kill her"—or that they were really disguised poison and we were trying to get rid of her. On those occasions we were called "the murderers." Or she may have believed that "the doctor told her not to take any more pills." Any and all excuses and wildly imaginative claims can be employed as patient avoidance of medications. It takes a creative caregiver to circumvent those excuses and claims to bring the loved one back around to readily accepting them.

As mentioned earlier, we'd frequently utilize Mary Belle's own phobias to accomplish this feat. We'd use her fear of constipation as our rationale. Since she wished to avoid that much-dreaded condition at all costs, we'd tell her that the pills would prevent it.

Each patient is different, as is each individualized circumstance. The caregiver is wisely guided to specific solutions by way of the patient's own particular psychological needs and/or mindset-of-the-moment. We've found that, oftentimes, the patient's highly irrational thought process surprisingly holds the key to a solidly rational solution.

Recognizing Signs of Anxiety

When our afflicted loved one exhibited signs of anxiety, her blood pressure would usually prove to be dangerously high when checked. Also, this physical condition would oftentimes evidence greater delusional events.

Although Mary Belle did indeed have an actual event with a severe nosebleed, and we had to call the ambulance to take her for cauterization, she later had the following delusional experience related to it.

One afternoon, when Sally was away from the cabin helping one of our neighbors with a wild animal rescue project, Mary Belle was sleeping in her living room recliner. From the office area where I was working I began hearing her talking in a highly distressed manner. I left the computer to check on her. She was sitting on the edge of her recliner and rocking back and forth in extreme agitation. She was holding her hands tightly over her nose. Profuse tears of pain and fear fell from her eyes as she began moaning about "this terrible pain" and cried out for someone to "please stop all the blood" and "please clean up the pools of blood on the floor!"

There was no blood.

She was not bleeding.

She'd been simply dreaming and had awakened to psychologically project that dream state image to the present reality.

I knelt in front of her and tried to make her see that there was no blood anywhere around. I showed her the clean fingers of her own hands. "See, Mary Belle? You're not bleeding. There is no blood anywhere. You were only dreaming. You were asleep."

She was so deeply into the delusion (or dream) that she could not be persuaded that it wasn't real and she continued to wail and cry about how badly she needed a doctor.

"When is the doctor coming?" she screamed in mounting hysteria. "Oh God! I need a doctor!" Her eyes lowered to the floor. Casting them over the spotless carpeting, she cried out, "Ohhh, God! Look at all that blood!"

Sally returned home at this point and immediately had me bring her the blood pressure monitor while she sternly talked to her mother about there being no blood and no nosebleed. The initial monitor reading came in at 202 over 165. Mary Belle was ready to stroke out on us. I ran for the medication while Sally had to literally shout at her mother in order to reach her.

The shouting worked.

The medication worked.

Finally, Mary Belle began to come out of her mental haze of hysteria and was greatly relieved to understand that she'd only been dreaming it all. Sally kept taking monitor readings until the pressure returned to a more acceptable range, and we all could finally relax a bit. Mary Belle was strongly cautioned to stay seated in her chair and, if she needed anything, we'd get it for her.

Delusional events and anxiety agitation can be triggers for dangerous health conditions. We'd come to learn that Mary Belle's blood pressure would be very high when she was having delusional or high anxiety/agitation events. Some signs of these events were the following behavioral traits:

1. Wringing of the hands
2. Pacing
3. Raking fingers through the hair
4. Constant deep sighing
5. Desperately trying to write down thoughts
6. Repeated unsuccessful attempts to verbally convey something that seems vitally important to the patient
7. A delusional event
8. Being blocked or prevented from doing something the patient is strongly compelled to do, such as "leaving" the property on sudden impulse. This leads to deep frustration causing the agitation.
9. Combativeness
10. Intensive frustration

If the caregiver can learn to become sensitively attuned to the patient's psychological state of being through perceptive observance of exhibited behavior (the first signs of growing agitation), then many times the potential for a serious incident occurring can be circumvented by quick responsive action. *Diversion of thought* is usually the first method of resolution the caregiver attempts, because diverting the patient's thought away from whatever is causing the agitation is most often the quickest way to prevent the event from escalating. In order to nip it in the bud, the caregiver must first recognize the presence of that bud of agitation. The following situation exemplifies one such successful utilization of the diversion of thought methodology.

One evening Mary Belle had taken paper and pencil to the dining table. She was desperately trying to get some tangled thoughts down on paper in some type of ordered format. It was clear that she wasn't achieving the desired goal and her frustration over this was causing growing agitation.

Sally went to the woodstove hearth where I had a stack of old manuscript papers ready to burn. She brought a handful over to the table where her mother sat.

"Mom? I know you're busy, but could you do something really important for us?"

Irritated over being interrupted, Mary Belle looked up at her daughter with a hard frown creasing her forehead. "What? What is it?"

"We need your help with something, Mom. It's really important."

The frown smoothed out. "You want me to help you with something?"

"Yes. We need your help with something we don't have the time to do ourselves."

The corner of Mary Belle's mouth tipped in pleasure. "I can help you out. I have time. What can I do?"

"Well, we need all the words on these pages that begin with S circled. We need to find a mistake and correct it. If you could just circle those we'll be able to find the error easier. It'd be a huge help to us."

Mary Belle shoved her own paper aside and took charge of the manuscript sheets. "I'll find the word for you. I can circle the S words."

As our patient set her mind to the new task at hand, the other piece of paper was slipped from the table and removed from her sight. She was so engrossed in her job that she'd completely forgotten all about what was so important for her to write down. Her state of growing agitation receded. You could almost hear the pounding blood pressure calm back down to a smooth and normal-flowing rate.

Every incident can't be caught by the caregiver because, if it were, that'd mean that the caregiver never takes her/his eyes off the loved one and that's just not reasonable. However, through *general* watchfulness and *overall* observation, the caregiver comes to recognize the individualized signs of growing anxiety/agitation in the patient's behavior. And the quicker these are circumvented through diversion of thought or other successful means, the easier life is for everyone.

Understanding vs Expectation

For the Alzheimer's caregiver, especially for the twenty-four-hour at-home caregiver, understanding this disease and its full range of symptomatic, clinical behavior is a lifesaving boon that removes all impulse toward having unrealistic or overly optimistic expectations, and then being sorely disappointed by same when reality hits the caregiver like the roar of an approaching whirlwind.

The fact of the matter is that this disease is one affecting the brain. It severely affects brain function and that means that one's afflicted loved one will not exhibit the same personality traits, attitudes, reasoning, and memory base as he/she always did prior to disease onset. As time passes, patient cognizance, rationale, general skills, and memory function deteriorate. Therefore, dealing with this disease is far different from caring for an individual with a physical impairment caused by a solely physical disease. With Alzheimer's, the caregiver cares for the mind in addition to the physical degeneration that ensues with the disease's progression. With this disease, the caregiver quickly learns that one's own personal understanding of the disease brings greater measures of inner strength required to maintain effective care for such a patient.

With Alzheimer's, the caregivers must clearly understand that they cannot *expect* to receive any of the following from their afflicted loved one: privacy, respect, kindness, courtesy, expressions of appreciation, personal freedom of movement, being believed, consideration, expressions of love, or any form of gratitude. What the caregivers do understand *receiving* from their patient are: juvenile responses such as name-calling and having the patient's tongue stuck out at you, being struck, lied about, having eyes on you all day, having someone listening to everything you say on the phone, being followed about, being expected to stand up to a barrage of verbal abuse, thanklessness, dirty looks, daily arguments over such things as when it's time to bathe, vindictiveness, etc.

Listing these traits and some of the commonly experienced situations associated with patient negativity isn't generated from an attitude of caregiver meanness or cynicism; it comes from hard-gained experience and a concerned attempt to provide potential future caregivers with an honest and solid sense of what this disease entails in regard to behavioral characteristics involved in patient-caregiver interaction.

If the patient is a loved one, such as a parent or significant other, the caregiver cannot be in any type of expectation as to the relationship continuing on in the status quo, *as it had up until that point in time.* To do so sets oneself up for a hard, disappointing fall. On the other hand, to understand that the patient will eventually develop a personality so different and seemingly polarized from what came before, and that the patient may indeed, then, appear to behave so uncommonly uncharacteristically of the person you once knew, makes for improved caregiving due to the tool of being armed with prior knowledge of the disease and all its behavioral ramifications.

Understanding that this adult patient is very much like a two-year-old, who throws temper tantrums, pouts, tells tall tales, and puts up fists in a knee-jerk response to frustration and anxiety, goes a long way in utilizing the qualities of having "mature rationale and no expectations" as effective management tools. Although the patient will exhibit an altered personality as the disease progresses, the wise caregiver also never forgets that this impaired individual is still her/his parent, spouse, or other long-loved individual. That unique and special relationship is the singular fact that can never be altered by the patient's behavior. No matter how much or how often the patient behaves in the manner of a complete stranger, the caregiver knows that there is a special bond-of-the-heart shared between them. And although the patient may have no recollection of that bond, the caregiver does. The caregiver still retains all the old, warm memories and still feels the warmth of love swirling within the heart.

Using Activities as Distraction

We've found that negative or high anxiety behavioral incidents can often be effectively deterred from quickly slipping into seriously combative events by distracting the patient's attention away from a specific subject matter that appears to be causing her/him anxiety or increasing agitation. Although there will be those frustrating times when no method of distraction will work, we have successfully managed to use this tool more times than I can count. Distracting the patient's single-mindedness by asking a totally off-the-wall question can also throw off the impending confrontational situation that the caregiver perceptively recognizes as developing.

One such example was when Mary Belle came up to me while nervously wringing her hands and began her anxiety-filled "man in the house" routine. Intentionally ignoring her voiced concerns, I looked her square in the eye and asked point blank, "Where'd you put that puzzle Tony sent you?"

"Puzzle? Tony?"

"Yes. Remember he sent you that cute puppy puzzle? I haven't seen it around anywhere. We should find it to make sure it's not lost."

"Tony's puzzle," she mumbled, turning to go in search of it. And the "man in the house" agitation fell off her like water off a mallard's back.

Distracting Mary Belle's focused thought from the delusional "bad man" in the house to a new thought associated with her loving son and his gift altered the entire aura of her personality and changed the whole situational configuration.

This incident took place at the time when Mary Belle could still comprehend and rationally respond to a question put to her. Yet, even when the disease progresses to the later stage when such understanding is far beyond the patient's cognizant capability, the use of springing a question on the patient can still prove effective. To the casual observer this type of verbal interaction will sound absolutely nonsensical, yet it doesn't matter, because nonsense has already become the patient's norm. To the patient, that silly conversation sounds perfectly logical. The following conversation is an example of such interplay.

Mary Belle was in her room and crying for her daddy. She was clearly working herself up into a growing state of agitation by pacing and raking her hands through her hair.

Beaming with a bright smile and speaking in an exaggeratedly cheery tone, Sally entered her mother's room. "Mother!" she loudly exclaimed to get her attention.

"Daddy?" Mary Belle asked.

"Laddie's over there," Sally responded while pointing to one of her mother's stuffed animals. "Laddie needs a nap. He's been up for a long time."

Mary Belle stopped crying and went over to the animal. Picking it up, she cooed while gently petting its head. "Such a sweet, sweet boy. He's a good boy."

"Why don't you rock him to sleep, Mother. I think he'd like that."

"What rock? The clock?"

"The clock on the wall shows that it's time for Laddie's nap."

"Cat's all gone now," Mary Belle mumbled. "No more cat." She looked up at Sally. "Where's your hat?"

"My hat's downstairs in the hall closet."

"You made a tall deposit?"

"Yes, Mother, I did it before it was time to give Laddie a nap. Aughhh, look at him. See how tired he is? He needs you to rock him to sleep now."

Again Mary Belle gave her attention to the tired little boy in her arms. "Yes, poor baby. You go on. I'm gonna rock Laddie to sleep now. Shhh."

Sally closed the door.

Mary Belle forgot about her previous upsetting thoughts of daddy as she fell asleep rocking Laddie in the warm, afternoon sunlight that spilled over her chair.

The Use of Activity as a Distraction

As illustrated, this activity doesn't have to be a difficult one. It can be something as simple as rocking a stuffed animal to sleep. It can be something as easy as searching for a misplaced sock or buttoning up laundered shirts. As long as the activity is well within the patient's ability to perform, it'll be a task that has the wonderful potential of distracting those frequently disturbing thoughts and successfully serve to avert a situation full of escalated anxiety and distress.

Eventually, Mary Belle reached the point where all rationale escaped her. Asking her the most simple question elicited a completely unrelated response. Yet there was always *something* within the context of that totally disconnected verbal exchange to catch her attention and divert her awareness away from a distressful idea and shift it toward a more constructive mental focus.

Sometimes the introduction of a new object will serve the same purpose. When the afflicted loved one is becoming visibly upset over a fixated thought, the caregiver can hold up an object—any object that's closest—and make some kind of declarative exclamation over it. The suddenness of this unexpected act seems to jar the patient out of his/her current woe. It pulls attention elsewhere and frequently serves to hold that attention in a cemented position that's far from the originating thought that instigated the initial signs of agitation. We once had Mary Belle sit in front of the picture window and gave her the important task of counting how many birds came to the feeders on the porch. This not only distracted her from a potential state of agitation, it also gave her that all-important sense of personal purpose—of accomplishing something productive in her long day.

Each caregiver will know the patient well enough to come up with individualized activities geared to their loved one's ever-changing personality and interests. It's not a difficult tool to employ. It's simple and, what's more, almost anything will serve as an effective distraction or manageable activity for the loved one to accomplish without frustration. The point is to achieve distraction of the patient's mental focus on a destructive or distressing thought. And as the disease progresses, the need for these distractions naturally becomes greater.

Ingenuity and a Pinch
of Basic Psychology

Ingenuity—that is, a little plain old creative imagination on the part of the caregiver—plays a huge role in effecting successful management of the Alzheimer's disease. As evinced by the various examples given in respect to the utilization of patient distraction, ingenuity is a valuable tool that comes equipped with multiple functions for multiple uses. The right tool for the right job, so to speak. It's the caregiver's trusty Swiss army knife that comes in handy in most all situations one finds oneself in.

An example of this use of ingenuity came from a neighbor friend of ours who was also an at-home caregiver for her mother. This woman's mother exhibited the same verbal communication difficulties as Mary Belle had during the beginning of her disease—that of not being able to successfully verbalize the right words to convey her precise thoughts or intentions. This afflicted woman fumbled and stumbled over her words in deep frustration, yet when speaking on the telephone, full sentences appeared to smoothly flow unhampered. Our neighbor's ingenuity led her to install an intercom system equipped with a handheld phone receiver for her mother to use. After this, they were able to maintain a higher level of communication between them for an extended period of time.

The above example of how a bit of extra thought applied to a patient-related behavioral or situational problem can result in unexpected and highly satisfying solutions is clear. However, the caregiver must *care* enough to expend the personal time and energy thinking through a problematic situation in efforts to glean resolutions. He/she must *want* to resolve them and expend the mental energy on analysis and possible solution options.

In an earlier chapter, I wrote about some of the difficulty we experienced coming up with appropriate activities for Mary Belle to occupy her idle time with. By "appropriate" I'm referring to activities geared to an adult's age, yet task-wise, simple enough for a small child to master without causing the undue stress of personal frustration or resulting in the patient's deepening sense of failure. We had somewhat of a difficult time locating the more simplified puzzles without juvenile images of cartoon characters depicted on them. We searched enough stores to eventually come up with acceptable scenic ones or those with baby animals as opposed to excessively juvenile images. First of all, we needed puzzles with fewer pieces, yet Mary Belle's mature age required corresponding age-related visuals. We didn't want to hurt her feelings or give her a sense that we perceived her as a child. That was important to us. Her continuing self-image was important for us to try to maintain because it was important to her. Although her behavior was indeed becoming more and more juvenile, we still strove to maintain her sense of elder dignity. So we solved the puzzle problem by taking the personal time to search stores for appropriate puzzles that would preserve her self-esteem and, at the same time, provide her with a sense of personal accomplishment.

Finding additional activities for her to occupy her idle time involved ingenuity and the use of a bit of psychology. We'd tried having her sort out her deceased husband's coin collection by dates, and that proved far too difficult for her to successfully manage. Therefore, the next logical step for us to take was to have her sort the coins by color. This, obviously, would've caused her to sigh and roll her eyes in indignation over the task's obvious simplicity, but after making an overdramatized show of "accidentally" dropping the bags of coins, we asked her if she would possibly help us re-sort the denominations which were now all impossibly mixed together. That simple solution completely altered her perception of the activity. It changed from one viewed as an obviously juvenile job to one of being productively helpful to us. The psychology of "accidentally" dropping the bags of coins on the floor was all that was needed to give her purpose, to give her something productive to do, and make her feel the sense of personal satisfaction that comes with doing something useful.

Another example of the situational use of ingenuity and basic psychology was unlocking the resolution for "incidents" by recognizing and allowing the patient's own rationale to provide the key to the solution.

An example of using the patient's own rationale was when we had to go after Mary Belle after she took off, striding purposely up the wooded drive for the purpose of "going home." She was single-minded. She wanted to "get out." She wanted to go to a nursing home where *they* would let her talk to her son "the moment" he called—talk to him without having to wait for Sally to finish her conversation with him first. We got her back to the cabin only after using her own rationale and telling her that she needed to go back to get her luggage.

Many times the patients themselves hold the key for an incident resolution within their own statements, behavior, or delusional episode. The delusion itself can provide the key that opens the escape hatch from it. All it takes is a little ingenuity and creative psychology to effectively utilize the key that's been offered.

Another way that ingenuity can come into play is through developing ways in which to effectively relieve patient confusion and forgetfulness. Since, on a daily basis or even as much as several times in one day, Mary Belle would forget where the bathroom was, it helped to make a large sign attached to the door that read, BATHROOM. To prevent her from accidentally letting the dogs out into the woods instead of into their dog yard, a sign was taped to the inside of the front door, WRONG DOOR. This worked like a charm. It worked in conjunction with placing another sign on the back door that said, DOG DOOR.

Such simple solutions. Yet they served to circumvent a host of problems.

When Mary Belle reached the later stage of the disease and, in the main, could no longer comprehend logical communications from others who addressed her, we found it expedient to perform tasks for her, instead of attempting to frustrate all involved by giving her directives that she couldn't understand. She would walk into the bathroom and turn in circles, forgetting why she'd gone into the room. If Sally or I noticed her doing this, we'd suggest that perhaps she went in there to use the bathroom. After hearing that, she wiped her dry hands on a towel. Then we'd say, "Don't you need to use the toilet?"

"Oh yes," came the reply before she sat down on the closed lid with clothing on.

"Mary Belle," we'd quickly say, "put the lid up first."

"You hid it?" she'd say.

"No, Mary Belle, the *lid*. Lift the *toilet* seat lid."

Then she'd reach for the sink faucet instead. There was no comprehension of what a toilet seat lid was. At this point, we'd enter the bathroom and lift the lid for her.

Yet, this wasn't enough, because she'd sit down with her slacks still around her waist.

"Pull your pants down, Mary Belle."

Instead, she'd begin fidgeting with her shirt buttons.

So you go to her and point to her slacks. "Your slacks. Pull down your *slacks* if you need to use the toilet."

"Yes, gotta use the toilet." And she'd again sit down fully clothed.

"No! Wait, Mary Belle!" And you'd have her stand up again. You'd tell her that she needed to remove her clothing if she intended to use the toilet, while placing your hands on the waist of the slacks and easing them down for her. Sometimes she'd become deeply indignant over your help. She'd already forgotten why you were doing it and react by slapping you in the face or pinching your arm. Yet, most times she'd thank you for the help and then go about using the facilities without further incident.

Making her bed was the same way. She couldn't understand why she shouldn't strip her bed five times a day. And if you asked her to please remake it, she couldn't manage the task. So you left the bed until the end of the day and then went in and did it yourself just before tucking her in for the night.

When her meals were eaten, and Sally or I would go into her room to collect her plate and utensils, these were rarely within view.

"Where's your plate, Mary Belle?"

"He told me to find my shoes," she'd reply.

"Your plate. Where is your dinner plate?"

"One . . . two . . . three. Here kitty-kitty," she called while clapping her hands for the imaginary pet.

"Let's look for your dinner plate, okay? Want to help me find your plate?"

She held up a sock. "Here."

"Here what? That's a sock."

"The mate. I found it."

"No, Mary Belle, not mate, your *plate.*"

"Here kitty-kitty."

So you decide that you've ridden the verbal merry-go-round long enough and don't say another word. Instead you busy yourself searching the entire room for that elusive dinner plate, plastic glass, and eating utensils. They may be anywhere. They may be scattered about in a shoe box, in a desk drawer, or between books on the bookcase. I once retrieved a missing plate—including her uneaten spaghetti—from inside her pillowcase.

So the most expedient move in situations like this was to enter the room and skip the questions regarding the plate's whereabouts and just go about searching for the vanished items yourself. On the surface, that didn't appear to be such an ingenious move, yet for the caregiver who has spent time attempting to elicit answers from someone who no longer comprehends the questions, avoiding the questions and doing for oneself becomes a saver of time and frustration.

Sharing Knowledge

The greater portion of the general public has little understanding of what Alzheimer's disease entails for the patient and caregiver. Most folks, when hearing the word *Alzheimer's*, automatically think of the clinical trait of forgetfulness as being the main symptom—sometimes the only symptom. They have no clear perception of the disease's broad symptomatic scope. Because of this tendency, they have no idea or comprehensive understanding of what an Alzheimer's caregiver goes through when caring for such a patient. This specific issue has been addressed in the many research books we studied. And, of course, we'd experienced it firsthand when we attempted to recount some of our experiences to our own friends, who appeared mildly uninterested because they didn't fully comprehend or appreciate what this type of caregiving entails.

Sharing knowledge of this disease with the patient's family, friends, and former business associates is an invaluable asset to helping these people come to a better understanding of what the afflicted individual is going through. In our case, we saw evidence of this wisdom when we initially began receiving disturbing calls from Mary Belle's relatives and friends. They were outraged over the poor care that Mary

Belle was allegedly receiving. Well . . . that happened because they didn't understand the nature of the disease. They didn't realize that it's common practice for these patients to tell tall tales, to make delusional statements, to relay half-truths, etc. After Sally spent hours and hours on the phone informing these people of the disease's behavioral characteristics, a couple of them deeply apologized for their misinformed and misdirected responses. They appreciated being apprised of the extent of the disease's behavioral characteristics. Others remained in doubt.

Knowledge is a wonderful thing. Knowledge is the greatest gift one can give another or even oneself. The Alzheimer's disease doesn't only equate to patient forgetfulness, it equates to an impressive host of other dramatic, behavioral alterations including, incredibly childish behavior, a loss of living skills, obsession and paranoia, possessiveness, abusive language, delusions, physical combativeness, hallucinations, fabrications, diminishing involuntary functioning of the body, and more.

Because the incidence of Alzheimer's is on the rise, people need to be informed as to its symptomatic characteristics. This information is not just for the immediate family members and close friends of those who are newly afflicted with the disease; it's for every adult human being living upon this planet who may, one day, begin to notice subtle signs of this disease appearing in their own behavior. This information is important for those who may, one day, be faced with the life-altering decision of taking on the task of themselves being an at-home Alzheimer's caregiver for one of their loved ones.

Human nature appears to display interest only in those subject matters that directly touch one's individual life or affect the singular quality of one's own personal space. Those issues which affect others seem to be of no particular interest or concern, yet these people don't perceive the possibility that, one future day, they too may be touched by such a disease. And then they (and theirs) will know nothing about it.

The idea for this book did not come to me because Alzheimer's has become a main issue to deal with in my life. The purpose of this book is not to talk about what we went through on a daily basis. It's not a personal issue. It's not about me. I didn't write it for self-serving purposes from a "poor us, look what we had to deal with" angle, nor did I write it for the purpose of gaining sympathy. I wrote it for the singular purpose of keeping my promise to Mary Belle to honestly document the characteristics of her specific disease in detail. Alzheimer's. She wanted her story told. This is just how it is. Plain and simple. It's just how it is.

The idea for this book came because I realized, on the whole, how many people don't understand what Alzheimer's is all about. The target group for this book is not specifically or uniquely the caregivers, nor the family and friends of patients; the target group is not even intended to be my own developed readership base . . . it's for the general public. By providing an in-depth look at how the disease affected and changed one woman and also at what that disease entails for the caregiver, I've endeavored to present a brutally honest accounting of what can be expected in terms of revealing the clinical elements of the disease.

This is a book that could've been titled: *Alzheimer's 101* or *Alzheimer's for Dummies*. It's meant to be presented in a simple manner yet, at the same time, be highly informative; a book uncloaking the mysteries of a disease every middle-aged person dreads coming down with and, consequently, is deathly afraid to look square in the eye.

In a casual conversation with a business associate and personal friend of mine, I once began to relay one of my particularly frustrating experiences with being a caregiver for this disease. The friend quickly cut me off with a condescending smile. "Oh, Mary," she sighed. "You of all people know that nothing's as bad as it seems. Everything takes care of itself." She didn't have to hit me over the head with her "cue" stick for me to hear what she was actually saying. I took her verbal cue. She didn't *want* to hear about it.

Once in a while an at-home caregiver needs a sounding board. This fact has been well documented in the Alzheimer's books over and over again. It's a lonely job, but as the caregivers soon discover, it gets even lonelier when they try to talk about it to those who are uninformed.

Knowledge

Knowledge of the disease is what the general public needs and requires for comprehensive understanding before they too discover a friend or family member suddenly finds themselves in desperate need of their understanding, and is heavily relying on them for heartfelt compassion and unflinching support. To hear "nothing is as bad as it seems," is to hear the voice of someone who's in denial, or someone who prefers not to become personally involved.

So my point is that honesty, as it's associated with the gaining of knowledge of this disease, must be a broadcast net. It must be utilized by everyone from the caregiver to the patient to the casual observer.

We were always honest with Mary Belle, in an attempt to maintain her understanding as related to what was happening to her. During the onset stage of the disease, when she had more lucid days than not, she'd become extremely frustrated with herself over her growing incidents of forgetfulness and increasing inability to precisely verbalize her specific thoughts.

Mary Belle knew she had the disease called Alzheimer's because we'd remind her of the fact. That fact helped to somewhat ease and assuage her deep frustration with herself. It gave a name to the reason for her personally unacceptable behavior. Initially, she'd requested books on the disease and we provided them by sharing some of our more basic reference volumes. She had some intelligent questions about its treatments and prognosis. We gave her the facts as we understood them. As she daily watched her capabilities slip from her grasp it seemed to help her to know that it was Alzheimer's disease that was causing this despised situation, not something that was "her fault."

Mary Belle was always a strong woman, ever the self-sufficient individual. She never wanted to be a burden to anyone and suddenly found that her former fears had been actualized in her elder years of life. Being openly honest and forthcoming with full information about her disease helped her acclimate to her environment here with us and gave her a reason as to what was happening to her. We sat and agreed with her that, no, it certainly didn't seem fair, yet the disease was a part of life as we now knew it and, as always, concluded with the assurance that we were all going to make the best of it by working together no matter how bad it got. This, of course, was a great comfort to her.

Sometimes, on the surface, being honest with full informational disclosure seems hard or harsh, but our experience has shown it to be a grounding factor for the patient who is trying so desperately to hold onto her/his rapidly diminishing identity, memory base, and basic living skills.

During the latter stages of the disease, when Mary Belle no longer understood much of anything that was said to her, there were times when we'd still remind her of the reason for why she couldn't manage to successfully make a bed or always remember to use the bathroom facilities. We could always tell by her behavior when this "reminding" would be effective. If she had a urinary accident in the middle of the room, and then sat around in the wet clothing until we discovered the mishap, then it was obvious that she had no awareness of what she'd done. These events were like those performed by someone with infantile awareness—knowing she'd done "something," but no recognition of any wrongness or inappropriateness associated with it. Yet, if she'd actually made some type of effort to *conceal* the accident by doing it behind a chair and then changing her clothing (or, more often, putting clean clothing over the soiled ones), then she clearly exhibited awareness and knowledge of her accident. In the latter case, reminding her of the disease-as-cause effectively helped to allay her sense of humiliation and/or guilt over the incident. "Mother," Sally would say in this case, "it's okay. You have a disease. The disease made you wet yourself instead of using the toilet. It's not your fault. Don't worry about it. We'll get you cleaned up."

Self-Knowledge

Knowing yourself. Knowing yourself by applying complete honesty when looking at your own inner feelings, attitudes, and perspectives. This is an invaluable tool for the effective caregiver. This is a valuable tool because, oftentimes, one's perspective of the disease can become mired down with personal attitudes which interfere with optimum levels of care. This is not to say that, by having these extraneous feelings, one has turned into a bad caregiver; it simply means that personalized attitudes and perspectives that shift off the mark hamper one's ability to provide care that is clear of unnecessary frustrations and stress factors.

For the Alzheimer's caregiver, rising and fluctuating levels of frustration are to be expected. They naturally come with the territory. However, frequently, these can be seen to be generated from a shift that's been made in the caregiver's personal attitude. And, this has a direct correlation to the "don't take it personally" factor mentioned earlier. As a caregiver for a loved one afflicted with this mentally debilitating disease, you have to stay focused on the primary fact that your patient is not "intentionally" misbehaving, at least not usually. *Brain dysfunction and the altering behavior it produces are not a voluntary choice of one's afflicted loved one.* This may sound simplistic and overly obvious to those unfamiliar with experiencing evidence of the disease on a routine basis, but it's not. The fact can easily slip into an emotionally compounded situation for a caregiver. Developing the habit of regularly analyzing one's attitudes and emotional responses is an activity that maintains the caregiver's perspective in a sharp and uncomplicated state. It serves to clear out the emotional pipes, so to speak. It keeps perspectives unclogged and washes away the slow buildup of those residual attitudes that cloud perceptual clarity. In fact, this practice is so vital to mental health that everyone should take the time to utilize it and reap its positive benefits. However, for the Alzheimer's caregiver, especially for the twenty-four-hour, at-home caregiver, this is a top priority activity that heads up one's To Do list.

Know yourself. Routinely take a good, hard look at how you've been responding to your patient's behavior. Check to see if you've been taking things far too personally. Dig around to discover why your frustration levels have increased or why your temper has dropped to such low combustion temperatures. Nobody ever said this was an easy disease to manage or care for. Even psychiatrists have mentors whom they're required to regularly consult for personal analysis. Giving yourself a routine emotional/attitude once-over is a tool well worth reaching for. Keep it handy—you'll need it at the most unexpected times.

Minimize Your Loved One's Fears

The Alzheimer's patients' minds are overflowing with all manner of fears. Some of these are way out front on the conscious level of awareness, while others are of the more hidden and subtle subconscious variety. They come in all shapes and sizes. Some of them become phobias. Some cause deep personal stress and anxiety. Others generate intensive agitation to the point of developing into full-blown physical combativeness. And some cry out for escapism measures. These are serious fears. They can't be idly dismissed as being frivolous or silly. They're not inconsequential to the patient. The patient's friends, family, and caregivers have a responsibility to understand the severity of this symptom. Although family and friends can sometimes alleviate these fears somewhat through light conversation or other diversionary tactics, it's ultimately up to the daily caregiver to keep a close eye out for any sign of the patient's falling, or plummeting, barometric fear reading.

When Mary Belle's anxiety rose in correlation with the lowering of the sun and she began exhibiting the hand-wringing and pacing associated with the sundowning syndrome, we'd either distract her attention from the windows or else take her out into the core of her fear, where she discovered that there was nothing there to be afraid of, especially when shown an approaching deer to marvel over or when we'd overdramatize our exclamations over the spectacular beauty of the mountain sunset. Shifting the sunset *anxiety* into a polarized experience of sunset *appreciation* most often served to circumvent instances of deepening inner stress and growing agitation due to the anticipated approach of nightfall.

The fear of being dropped off at a nursing home every time we took Mary Belle anywhere was alleviated by applying reverse psychology—by *increasing* the frequency of her outings. In this manner, the more she went out somewhere in the car and saw that the dreaded drive didn't end up at a nursing home destination, the deeper her trust became. The greater the trust, the lesser the fear and related anxiety. Sally would take her mother for a leisurely drive through the mountains and they'd stop at various places along the way to take in the beauty of the various scenic vistas. Mary Belle would accompany her daughter on errands involving short trips here and there. Eventually, when the disease progressed and Mary Belle couldn't be trusted to not open the car door when the vehicle was in motion or suddenly grab at the steering wheel, her fear of being taken to a nursing home vanished altogether because, at that point, the idea of taking leisurely drives had been hit out of the ballpark. There were no more drives, unless they were necessitated by a visit to the doctor's office for a checkup, or stitches, or a fast-track ride down to the hospital emergency room, when I would accompany them to keep a close watch on our distressed or injured passenger, while Sally concentrated on the driving.

The delusional fear that we were starving her dog was taken out of the picture when Mary Belle's rational behavior diminished to the point of permanently relocating her into her "little apartment" upstairs. At that time, whenever her dog was up with her, we'd too frequently find the dog in a nearly strangulated position of having a bathrobe sash tied to her collar and tightly wrapped around the leg of the bed. Molly was a devoted animal. There was never any reason to tie her anywhere for the purpose of keeping her near Mary Belle. Yet, as time passed and our patient began mistreating the dog, Molly began to show signs of fearing her mistress and she'd avoid going upstairs to be with her. Molly would actually run and hide in an effort to avoid being with Mary Belle. Molly was exhibiting neurotic animal behavior.

So the overall solution was to send Molly off to Tony in North Carolina. Tony loved his mother's dog and was more than willing to take her into his home. Mary Belle never missed her dog's presence. Mary Belle never realized that her dog no longer lived in the household with us. And never again did she experience woe over Molly being starved. The solution came down to one of being an out of sight, out of mind resolution.

Prioritizing Behavior

On the surface, it would perceptually appear that, for the twenty-four-hour at-home caregiver, all forms of behavior evinced by an afflicted loved one should be classified as Priority One. However, upon closer examination of the various types of behavior, the tendency to perceive all behaviors as belonging within the confines of this singular category classification is revealed as being a false assumption. It could even be viewed as being an "alarmist" type of idea, for many types of behavior can be taken with nothing more than that proverbial grain of salt. In actuality, some behaviors don't even deserve that grain of salt attention because many of them have no possible potential of producing harmful effects or outcomes. Therefore, they can be completely ignored altogether. And, what's more important, an alarmist caregiver is not an effective caregiver. An alarmist caregiver will intensify a situation by invariably exacerbating the patient's behavior and state of mind.

The Alzheimer's patient's behavior is so incredibly diverse that the wise caregiver views that wide range with a sharp eye toward behavioral triage, much like the triage nurse in a hospital emergency room does. Assessment. The patient's behavior is assessed according to either its potential for causing *imminent physical harm* or its potential for *increasing the patient's emotional agitation* and, therefore, quickly creating an escalated, physically combative incident. While there is clear evidence of these two possible outcomes being of the *Priority One* variety, most others fall into a placement somewhere below that critical level.

The at-home caregiver cannot afford to be an emotional reactionary. One's tendency to overreact to every observed behavioral incident will only result in the caregiver causing him/herself to become a Type A personality, full of self-imposed, undue stressors in life. For example, the patient's act of secreting a steak knife in the pocket of her/his clothing does not warrant the same caregiver response as when that same patient strives to conceal a postage stamp purloined from one's desk. The former requires immediate action. The latter can be ignored without consequence. For the caregiver to get hyper and make a scene over a postage stamp is an unnecessary response that will only lead to further discord and patient agitation—possibly leading to a combative situation. It will only exacerbate a purely innocuous incident. Keeping one's cool through the use of clear perspective toward prioritizing various behaviors is a tool the caregiver uses so often that it becomes second nature.

When Mary Belle banged on her wall for hours on end, we left her alone because, eventually, she tired of the activity and turned her attention elsewhere. However, if she was banging on her television screen or the window glass with a hard object such as a ceramic figurine, then that obviously was behavior that required immediate attention.

Assessing each type of behavior with an eye to priority serves to maintain a more even keel to one's day, especially the caregiver's. When Mary Belle would take it in mind to walk out the cabin door and stroll up the drive, we wouldn't overreact by immediately racing after her. We'd observe her through a window to see if her intent was to merely go for a short stroll for the purpose of getting a little fresh air and exercise, or for the purpose of taking off into the woods with the single-minded goal of getting to her imaginary shoe factory job. If she appeared to be simply enjoying being out in the pleasant weather, then we'd leave her alone. On the other hand, if she began striding further up the drive, we'd have to take appropriate measures to insure that she remained on the property and didn't wander up to the road or get lost in the forest.

Prioritizing behavior gives your loved one some lifestyle space and leeway. It provides him/her with greater measures of that all-important sense of independence. Who cares if they're ripping pages out of a magazine? What harm does that cause? After the first time that happened, you will probably put away those special magazines you want to preserve and only leave out the ones that you'll eventually end up tossing away after a time anyway. By the way, old merchandise catalogs are great magazines to keep on hand, because an Alzheimer's patient who's in the latter stages of the disease can no longer read (comprehend) magazine articles, and the catalogs, loaded with a vast array of diverse and colorful "things to look at," can occupy hours of their time. These, as opposed to those periodicals full of wordy articles, will hold their attention far longer.

Verbal abuse from the patient fits neatly into this important caregiver's tool category. It's admittedly upsetting and emotionally hurtful for an adult child to hear a parent calling them all manner of names or vilely spitting out a string of obscenities at them, yet that's the most important and effective time to keep your cool by recalling the old adage that that same parent reminded you to remember when you yourself were a youngster. Remember? Sticks 'n' stones? A caregiver is going to voluntarily take on all manner of unnecessary emotional luggage if he/she internalizes these patient verbal expressions and turns them into a personal matter.

When one of us brought Mary Belle a hot meal and she looked down at it with a smirk and sarcastically spouted, "I'm not eating that rotten stuff. You're just trying to kill me, you Snot/Slut." We'd only respond to that by cheerily exclaiming something like, "Look, Mary Belle! All your favorite foods! There's fresh-baked cheesecake for dessert when you're done eating this." And then leave the food on her table for her to ponder. No response is given in reaction to the name-calling or the mention of the food being "rotten." No attention is even warranted to those negative elements of the verbal exchange.

The wise caregiver gets to the point where the patient's mean statements aren't even heard anymore. Why is that wise? It's wise because if the caregiver responds with, "That's not nice. You're being mean. You hurt my feelings by saying those things to me after I just prepared a good meal for you," then the patient is immediately drawn into an extended opportunity for response—and it's usually further abusive comments that ultimately deepen the entire situation.

Remember, the patient is your loved one. Granted, there are times—many times— when you have to remind yourself of that fact. But that fact will never change. Yet, what's even more important to remember is the reality that that loved one has a disease affecting the mind's thought process. Therefore, the very special relationship that once strongly existed between you is no longer a shared one—has suddenly, seemingly overnight, become one-sided. It's the *caregiver's* side that maintains that bond of love and devotion. The patient's side has fallen down long ago. A good perspective for a caregiver to have regarding this concept is to view their loved one's love and memory of the former relationship they shared as being the last, lone autumn leaf that has finally been blown from the Tree of Love by the bitter winter winds. Or perhaps liken it to the woodland bear that hibernates, shifting all elements of its former awareness into a suspended state of sleepfulness. The patient's awareness of all former familial bonds and emotional relationships slips into an ever-deepening state of sleep. And for the caregiver who is left holding her/his end of that relationship up . . . love never falls asleep.

It never even nods off.

Not even for a moment.

Conceptually, the prioritizing tool is closely associated to the issue of parenthood. When a couple become parents for the first time, the baby is handled with kid gloves. The child is watched like a hawk for any signs of illness, bottles and toys are meticulously sterilized, and the child is followed about the house when the youngster begins toddling around and exploring the world, etc. Yet, after several babies have come this couple's way, the bottle sterilization process loses its former sense of urgency, the common cold is taken with a grain of salt as it's cared for, the child's bumps and spills are more likely to be brushed off with administering a soothing kiss and cartoon bandage instead of panicking and rushing the bellowing child off to the nearest emergency room. The parents become more relaxed and less uptight with anxiety. They've learned to prioritize events, illnesses, and situational events in their children's lives. They rarely overreact anymore. They've gained a natural skill for triage.

So then, if your Alzheimer's loved one becomes physically combative when you attempt to remove her/his street clothes at night and put her or him into sleepwear when it's time for bed, why continue putting each other through such an exhausting experience? What's the harm in someone sleeping in her clothing? Well, yes, society has this ideological concept that the practice isn't hygienic or socially proper, yet the Alzheimer's patient no longer gives a thought to such inconsequential mores. Sleeping in one's street clothing is an issue that's so low on the priority list that it trails miles behind all the issues that come before it. So you go ahead and just let your loved one sleep in whatever pleases her. Creating a scene over such innocuous events proves foolish and unnecessary.

When Mary Belle dressed herself (or decided to change her "night" street clothing) in the morning and donned five shirts, we left her alone. We left her alone because the alternative of making her remove four of those shirts just wasn't worth the physical fight to get it accomplished. Besides, five minutes later she'd have them back on again. So, the caregiver ignores those five shirts in the first place and everyone stays calm. The avoidance of fighting over the number of shirts equated to an avoidance of having a highly agitated loved one.

Prioritizing is a "mellowing-out" process for the caregiver. You might even say it's taking a "whatever" attitude toward your loved one's odd behaviors. If the behavior doesn't carry the potential to cause anyone harm, then what harm is that behavior? Though, for sure, that behavior may be socially unacceptable to most people, or perceived as being extremely odd, or out of character for most people, it can be overlooked because, for an Alzheimer's patient, that type of behavior *is* normal. And the sooner the caregiver recognizes that reality and accepts it, the smoother life will be for everyone involved.

Routine

Routine is an invaluable tool benefiting both the patient and the caregiver for the maintenance of a fairly stable emotional state in the patient's life. Routine reinforces a sense of predictability in the patient's day and lessens his/her incidents of rising anxiety and the potentialities to experience various fears of the unknown.

Through our own experience we've observed that the Alzheimer's patient is most comfortable and generally calm when she/he isn't exposed to an overly altered daily routine. Thoughts of having to interact with visiting company and the expectation of having to be social can be a trigger for fear. This is closely related to the psychological symptoms of what's commonly known as social anxiety, where a multitude of fears surface: fear of being unable to verbally communicate adequately, fear of embarrassing oneself in front of others, fear of strangers invading one's personal home space, fear of someone coming to take the patient away to a nursing home, etc.

Everything that tends to support the patient's sense of comfort and normalcy is a plus when attempting to keep those fears at bay. Daily routines help give the patient stability in life and offer a more solid sense of connectedness to reality. Her expectation of being handed that first cup of coffee in the morning and that same act being actualized when it's followed through helps to start the day off normally. Tucking her into bed every night and turning on the night light offers a sense of security and helps to allay her night fears.

Caregiver consistency offers one's afflicted loved one a sense of stability and an invaluable lifeline to the reality that she finds slowly and insidiously slipping away with each passing day. At times, this sense of routine is the singular straw to grasp for in an attempt to hold on to the remaining threads of her former life. It creates a feeling of dependability. Solidity within an ever-changing world that's quickly closing in around her. A stepping stone of terra firma amid the new swirling stream waters that seem to be quickly rising over her mental shoes.

For Mary Belle, having her dog with us was her main lifeline to stability. Molly kept her grounded. The pet kept her routinely focused on an aspect of consistency in her life. And that served her well until she reached the latter stages of the disease when recognition of individuals (and old family pets) slipped away into the unknown mists of the mind.

During this former time when Molly was a vitally important element in Mary Belle's life, our own routine greatly helped to stabilize her days. She could count on getting up in the morning and silently sitting around with us in the living room with our "wake-up" cups of coffee. She could count on receiving three meals a day. Whether she actually ate them was another issue, but at least she knew regular meals would be provided and placed before her. This "food" factor may sound far too simplistic to most people, but for the Alzheimer's patient, anxiety over not having enough food in the house is a frequent source of personal paranoia.

Letting Mary Belle carry around her address and telephone list of friends and relatives was an incredible comfort to her. This was a great source of stabilization, because she perceived that list as her ongoing physical connection to those she knew and loved in her life. To her way of thinking, the physical act of carting the list around with her was the same as holding those people's hands. It was her way of keeping in constant touch with each person on the list. Although she'd frequently become obsessive about the list, especially if she'd misplaced it, the stapled pages continued to provide her with a soothing sense of security and gave an added aspect to her idea of routine. It helped to maintain her sense of groundedness. As with her dog, eventually Mary Belle's interest in the address list fell by the wayside. She could no longer connect visual memories to any of the names she read. She reached a point when no name rang a bell and all the individuals listed became complete strangers. The importance of the list was finally lost on her. And only then did routine also lose its value as a useful caregiver tool.

Recognizing the Importance of Your Patient's Possessions

It doesn't take the mind of a physicist to understand that the personal possessions of Alzheimer's patients are deeply comforting for them to be surrounded by. Upon the most cursory observation, it's obvious that these possessions have taken on a much greater and more important role in the afflicted individual's life than mere possessiveness of material goods; they solidly equate to stability, to having roots (groundedness), and security in a world that appears to be shrinking the patient's sense of confidence, with the encroachment of more and more insecurities making appearances within each passing week.

Conceptually, the Alzheimer's patients' behavioral responses that are associated with their personal possessions can be closely linked to the same psychological elements related to the ragged security blanket that toddlers tightly clutch to their small chests. When the toddler has that blanket firmly grasped in hand, not giving a care to its tattered and soiled condition, the child has that reassuring sense that all is right with her/his world. Without it, frustration, anger, irritation, anxiety, and fear can gain a quick hold.

Sometimes the patient's possessions, even a singular one having special meaning, will be the only tie to reality the patient has to hold on to.

When Mary Belle saw her personal things on our living room book shelves, in the china hutch, and in kitchen cupboards, she felt a rooted sense of belonging—of truly belonging somewhere. She felt that this was her home, too, not just Sally's and mine. It provided her with reinforcement and she shed her feeling of being a transient in a temporary living situation. Her possessions placed about the cabin served to reinforce our continual verbal assertions that indeed "this is *her* home too, that she is no mere visitor here." Her possessions converted to an ideology that underscored her right to be here and that she was not going to be going anywhere else. They were her anchor of security in a churning sea of change and unpredictability.

Mary Belle's various types of behaviors clearly reflected this philosophy whenever she got it into her head that she wanted to die. In that case, she immediately turned to her possessions as a first response to her recurring dark idea. It was her possessions she thought about. It was her possessions that began to get amassed in various piles on her bed for the purpose of disbursing to friends and family as bequeathed gifts. It didn't seem to matter to her if those personal items were her underwear or the trash from her wastepaper basket because, in her mind, they were all her possessions. That fact was the bottom line. And that activity of hers exemplified how her possessions were directly associated with her own idea of beingness, of being connected to the physical world reality—to home, family, and friends.

Having personal possessions serves as security to the Alzheimer's patient, especially family photographs around one's room. They provide comfort and stability. Both act as aids to alleviate a multitude of phobias related to aloneness, to being uprooted from familiar surroundings and, perhaps, even to being sent to a nursing home.

When Mary Belle first came to live with us, she had a deep fear of missing the acknowledging of her friends' birthdays. To circumvent this fear we took out our own calendar and recorded each of her personal friend's special days. In this manner, she could go over to the calendar whenever she wanted (as much as ten times a day) and see when one of her friend's birthdays was approaching. This comforted her, and one less fear was present for her to contend with. Eventually, as time passed and Mary Belle's disease progressed, she gave no more thought to people's special days of remembrance. That was when we began keeping track of them for her. We'd purchase the gift for her to send and then help her sign her name to the greeting card. However, when the recipient received the gift and called to express appreciation, Mary Belle wouldn't recall sending anything and responded with animated surprise. She'd exclaim with sentiments similar to the following, "I didn't *know* it was your birthday!" Shooting one of us a hard, menacing glare, she'd add, "Nobody *told* me!" Her friends quickly got the message that Mary Belle's memory was failing far quicker than they'd thought. When they got back on the telephone with Sally, they thanked her for sending off the gift and expressed their understanding of the situation. Usually, they'd be sympathetic and suggest that Sally not bother with the additional work of maintaining her mother's gift list. They didn't want to burden her further by having her sending presents in her mother's stead, that Mary Belle herself no longer had memory of sending. Everyone thought it pointless once the disease reached that stage.

When Mary Belle no longer had any concept of time or holidays associated with the changing seasons, we still maintained her list for her. Because she carted it around so much and made nonsense notations all over it, Sally had to reprint a fresh copy of it from the computer at least twice a month. She used a large type, so it was easier for her mother to read. Although Mary Belle lost her sense of time and date and didn't equate those dates on her list to related actual birthdays to remember, the list was still a continuing source of comfort and stability for her. It was one of her primary sources of grounding connection to those who were familiar to her. The list allayed most sensations of aloneness that had the potential to sweep over her like a weighted, emotional shroud. Like her personal possessions, the list became another form of security blanket to clutch to her breast. This held true until the disease progressed into its latter stage when all the recognition and memory of family members or friends were lost forever.

The caregiver soon learns which of the patient's personal possessions are perceived as powerful and effective shields against fear and understands their great importance. These then serve as highly prized tools for helping to reinforce the patient's sense of belonging and security.

Tools so simple, yet so very, very invaluable.

Acceptance

Although the patient subliminally benefits from the utilization of acceptance as a tool, it's the caregiver who reaps the most value from its consistent use. Acceptance provides a barrier, surrounding the caregiver, that protects her/him from receiving damaging emotional wounds. Being around someone who continually makes faces at you or never believes anything you say, being exposed to someone who calls you names and tells lies about you can be emotionally unnerving to say the least. It can wear down the fabric of your resolve to a tattered and threadbare state. Acceptance keeps this fabric in a pristine condition. It's like spraying Scotch Guard over one's fragile sensitivities. Acceptance creates a protective "personal space" between you and incoming psychological missiles that serves to neutralize the damaging effects of another's thoughtlessness or mean-spirited comments.

Understanding Alzheimer's symptomatic clinical behavioral characteristics and having the corresponding acceptance of those traits creates a natural barrier—a neutral zone, if you will—for the caregiver who is continually exposed to psychological negativity and physical combativeness from the patient, especially if that patient is a loved one.

Accepting the fact that the caregiver isn't going to be shown any signs of appreciation or gratitude for all he/she does for his/her loved one is a major element of providing good and effective care. Remaining neutral about abusive language directed at or about you is part and parcel of dealing well with the disease in an effective manner. Letting negativity roll off the skin of your sensibilities is one of the caregiver's most useful tools for insuring self-preservation and the maintenance of an emotionally level day.

Having acceptance doesn't mean that the caregiver slips into an apathetic attitude and resorts to completely ignoring the patient. That's not acceptance, that's denial. In that case, it's not caregiving, it's evidence of an inability to "deal" with the job. Sometimes there can appear to be a fine line between exhibiting the shining beauty of true acceptance and the shadowy grotesquesness of apathy. The conscientious caregiver keeps a sharp eye on where their position is being maintained in relation to that all-important and revealing line.

Throughout my lifetime I've included a considerable amount of philosophical material devoted to the subject of acceptance within my published works. I've done this because I can't ever overstress the importance of gaining this invaluable and precious "Quality of Perspective." Having acceptance serves one well throughout one's entire lifetime, not only when or if you have to one day deal with caring for a loved one afflicted with Alzheimer's disease, but in all possible life situations and types of interactive relationships that one finds oneself in. Acceptance greatly lessens the often devastating effects of deep disappointments, unreached goals, unexpected turns of events, the potentially hurtful behavior of others, etc. I liken acceptance to having gained a greater measure of maturity in life, a maturity directly related to overall perspective. It acts like oil over troubled waters, to smooth out the emotionally choppy waves of life. It is invaluable in providing a source of inner serenity amid turbulence and chaos. Having acceptance curbs impulsiveness and overreaction, it holds back the urge toward expressing those knee-jerk reactions—wisely keeping them in check.

Acceptance says, "I'll hold judgement and response until I've taken the time to thoroughly examine all aspects of this situation." And, more importantly, it says, "I gracefully accept every life situation, event, and behavior of others that I know have no possibility of being changed." Therefore, acceptance allows one to more readily and easily roll with the punches that can seemingly come out of nowhere. It lets one ride with the current instead of continually struggling against its unbeatable force.

These ideologies are never so clearly exemplified as when one's life situation has suddenly become inexplicably intertwined with the disease of Alzheimer's for, of itself, the disease presents a myriad of opportunities for the afflicted one's family members and friends to practice the grace of acceptance.

Calmly accepting the mean-spirited verbal statements directed at you from your loved one as merely being one clinical behavioral characteristic of the disease is having the grace of acceptance. Your immediate response to these is not one of knee-jerk anger, personal affront, hurt, verbal retaliation, or chastisement. It's simple acceptance, where no response at all is given because you allow the unkind words to quickly roll off your slick back and let them swiftly flow away into the stream of forgetfulness.

Acceptance is the best aid for the caregiver's tool of not taking things personally. Those mean-spirited words flung at you or the physical strike from your loved one is never taken personally when acceptance has taken up permanent residence in your heart. This is because you know it's the disease doing these things, not your loved one. Your loved one, if in full possession of their former mental faculties, would be absolutely mortified to know they had been behaving in such an uncharacteristic and unloving manner. Therefore, acceptance also brings the additional grace of compassion to the fore of one's perspective when interacting with someone afflicted with this particular disease. Understanding that the patient would normally be deeply humiliated and embarrassed by routinely exhibiting such unkind behavior goes a long way in accepting the fact that now their mind has irretrievably lost the capability of grasping that recognition. They reach the point where they're no longer culpable or held responsible for the actions generated from a mind without social scruples or behavioral conscience. Acceptance of that fact goes a long, long way toward providing effective care that greatly benefits both the patient and the caregiver.

Dispensing the Magical
Properties of the Humor Elixir

When an Alzheimer's caregiver has a good and well-exercised sense of humor, that individual has a handful of sparkling gold dust—a veritable treasure that sprinkles one's day with shimmering, golden particles of amusing anecdotes to laugh about. That precious sense of humor has the potential of magically transforming a deep sigh of frustration into a quick chuckle, a down-turned frown into a broad smile, and mysteriously altering a potentially explosive, combative situation into one of calm and laughter.

Its properties are soothing and take immediate effect.

They go down easy.

Discovering Mary Belle's final diagnosis sent Sally and me on a research quest that not only reached out along the shelves of various bookstores, but also to the various Internet sites related to the disease. Sally came across one that served as a caregivers' support site and viewing the humor employed by the participants was a surprising delight to see.

Daily (and nightly) caregiving for an individual afflicted with this particular disease can frequently plummet one into the shadowed regions of deep frustration and even into the shadows of depression. Just the basic nature of the disease creates a thankless situation for such caregivers and, as all the reference books on the disease clearly point out with great emphasis, those healthcare aides *need* emotional support.

One particular interactive Net site invited Alzheimer's caregivers to come up with their own experiential "stages" of the disease. One individual named a stage: *The Throwing Garbage Out a Closed Window Stage.* There were many other funny entries as well.

To be truthful, when I first saw this and was yet of the uninformed opinion that it wasn't nice to make fun of others, especially those with a disease, I thought these people were being mean and excessively cruel to make that kind of fun of their Alzheimer's patients' behaviors. Yet, after experiencing life as a fulltime at-home caregiver for over three and a half years, I realized that the routine use of humor was a wonderful management tool—general management of both the patient and the caregivers' own mental health. I realized that those Net site folks weren't actually making fun of their patients. Oh, no, they weren't doing that at all; they'd found a wildly effective way to lighten up their frustrating experiences and laugh at their own responses to those unpredictable, ongoing events. I realized that, more than anything, they weren't laughing and poking fun at their patients, but, more accurately, were laughing at each other as they openly shared their experiences and offered other caregivers useful suggestions for behavioral problem-solving techniques. For those people, sharing experiences was invaluable, and the act of utilizing humor was as priceless as their continuing support for one another.

We, too, have found the prized benefits of using humor as a means of safeguarding one's mind (emotional stability) and heart (wounded feelings) when dealing with an Alzheimer's patient. If you can laugh at something, that "something" doesn't have a chance in hell of turning into a hurtful element. This does not mean that the caregiver goes around audibly laughing at everything. It simply means that, psychologically, humor becomes a tool of perspective, with which the patient's behavioral events take on a much lighter slant and tone.

For example, when Mary Belle stuck her tongue out at one of us, Sally or I could have reacted by internalizing the act and taking it personally, thereby causing ourselves to experience hurt feelings, or just ignore the behavior and inwardly think it was wildly humorous. We didn't visibly grin back at the patient in response. We didn't make a demeaning or chastising comment to Mary Belle. And we certainly didn't laugh in her face. We just acted as though we didn't see her do it and then mentally made light of it.

Much of the most effective Alzheimer's caregiving response is "looking the other way"—ignoring and not adding fuel to a potentially flammable situation by negatively responding in a like juvenile manner. There are many behaviors one can overlook and ignore. These are the harmless, childish acts that the patient will increasingly display as the disease progresses. If you respond to these by returning behavior through negative responses, or by coming unglued, or showing similar types of reactions, the patient will then identify his/her own childish behaviors as being "one of your buttons." No, no, you don't want to give them more of your buttons to push, because they probably have enough of them pegged already.

When Mary Belle returned home with us from an evening of swimming at the health club, and we all discovered that she'd put her underwear on over her slacks, we all laughed and made a big joke of it instead of turning it into an issue she should be reprimanded for and be embarrassed about. By making light of it, Mary Belle's embarrassment over the situation was turned into a funny event she shared with us, and we all had a good laugh. The amusement of the behavior far outshone the humiliation she could've experienced. Chastising patients for this type of typical behavior is fruitless and unproductive toward accomplishing the goal of maintaining a good ongoing relationship.

Sometimes when Mary Belle came to me with her hand-wringing story of that "man in the house," I'd turn to her with a big smile and teasingly say, "Well go *get* him! Go ask him for a *date!*" And suddenly, as if by magic, my unexpected comment would cause the anxiety-filled lady to break out laughing. So, instead of spending hours on end trying to convince her that there was no man in the cabin, the situation quickly ended up on a humorous note rather than one heavy with deepening fear. This is not to imply that one's fears are laughable, but humor can oftentimes turn the tables on some types of imaginary or unfounded fears.

Humor . . . the magical elixir.

No prescription needed.

Reach for it often.

IV. TAKING THE STING OUT OF CAREGIVER GUILT

The Caregiver's Golden Right to Identity

The Alzheimer's Backlash Phenomenon of Caregiver Guilt

Guilt.

The subject of this entire section is guilt. Caregiver guilt. To be more precise, caregiver *false* guilt. And it is the rare general information book on Alzheimer's that fails to address this highly recognized issue, as it's specifically associated with the primary care-provider for a loved one afflicted with the disease. Why? Because unlike the caregiving elements associated with other types of diseases, guilt appears to be a strong residual *symptom* that the *caregiver* vicariously contracts. It seems to be a natural "effect" based on the "cause"—that cause being a patient with increasing dementia. When that patient is a loved one, the degree of guilt evidenced has a direct correlation to the depth of that love. The greater the love, the greater the guilt—false guilt.

I'm not talking about or implying that the Alzheimer's caregiver experiences guilt caused by providing inadequate or poor quality care. This is not at all what this guilt is related to, because the fact is, the higher the quality of care, the deeper the guilt. I'm referring to the type of guilt associated with the caregivers' emotional responses to providing that excellent and attentive care. Why, you might wonder, would a caregiver possibly experience any guilt over giving excellent care? Let's look at some of the facts associated with this well-documented phenomenon.

This book is primarily focused on the at-home, twenty-four-hour caregiver, that is, the caregiver who lives every hour with a patient whose behavior is abusive, demanding, defiant, childish, physically combative, irrational, unpredictable, etc. Essentially, the at-home caregivers have chosen to devote an unspecified portion of their lives to caring for a loved one who may or may not even recognize them as such—as being their daughter, son, or life companion. This caregiver has accepted and voluntarily shouldered the heavy responsibility of providing a loved one with a familiar and secure environment, taking on the responsibility of protecting that loved one from doing personal harm to her/himself, taking on the burden of making sure that that loved one receives proper daily medication and medical treatment, handling that patient's financial obligations, providing activities and entertainment, etc. In essence, the at-home caregiver has accepted the fact that she has voluntarily set aside her own personal life for an undetermined block of time (usually several years) in deference to devoting that time to the care of a loved one.

The caregiver's time has suddenly become filled with hours of alternating between a multitude of occupational hats—the hats of nurse, psychologist, servant, accountant, social director, maid, chauffeur, cook, waitress, personal secretary, and more. The caregiver's own life shifts into the shadows and, week by week, becomes lost in the shuffle as more and more time is taken up with dealing with the patient's medical care, social activities, and business obligations. But, most of all, time is taken up with being drawn into the patient's vacillating emotionality of the deepening dementia. And, this is where the caregiver guilt enters in.

Although the caregiver dearly loves her patient, whether that patient be mother, father, or other cherished relative, being exposed to the dementia of Alzheimer's on an hourly basis, day after day and night after night, wears on the caregiver's psychological and emotional fabric. It can't be stressed strongly enough that this is not an issue of the caregiver's self-absorbed ego, whereby its sense of self-importance conflicts with the new shift-of-attention to another. *The wearing down of the caregiver's emotional fabric has nothing to do with ego or selfishness.* And that statement is the crux of the guilt, for the caregiver will feel as though she/he is being selfish by having negative thoughts, reactions, or feelings toward the patient, or experiencing moments of regret. These caregiver "feelings" are such a strongly recognized attachment to Alzheimer's disease that new Alzheimer's caregiver support groups are being established nationwide as fast as mountain wildflowers suddenly appear after a gentle spring rain.

So, what types of "feelings" are we talking about here? Some of the "guilt chapters" in the Alzheimer's reference books that Sally and I had read at the outset detailed caregiver thoughts that ranged from regrets over taking on the job to feelings that verged on a "death wish" for their patient: *"Please God, Dad's mind is gone. He doesn't recognize anyone anymore. He can't do a thing for himself without help. I'm so tired. Please take him into your arms tonight."* Although Sally and I had never experienced thoughts or feelings of guilt that reached those proportions, I believe the best way to convey this concept is through our own personal experiences with it.

Folks who know Sally and myself on a personal basis would not ever say that we're selfish individuals. In my opinion, Sally is one of the most giving persons I've ever known. If she hears that someone is in need of something she has, she'll give it away without thinking twice about it. Once, after she left the cabin to go pick up the mail in Cripple Creek and was driving along our twisting mountainside roads, she happened to pass by a lone Department of Transportation worker, who stood beside his truck and seemed to be deeply confounded as to how he was going to load some scrap railroad ties into it all by himself. Sally told me that it was as if she could read his thoughts, so clear were the combined elements of the young man's body language. So, she pulled off onto the shoulder to offer him some assistance. While she was helping the young man, he kept repeatedly asking her, "Lady, why are you doing this?" And she simply kept echoing, "Because you looked like you needed some help." As they loaded up the ties, the man continued shaking his head in disbelief over the good fortune that had come his way. I used this story as a prime example that reflects the sorry state our society has slipped into. It clearly exemplified how puzzled folks become when a complete stranger stops to help them out—without first being asked or paid to do so. But, then, that's the kind of person my friend is. Neither of us is afraid of work or of spontaneously offering to help someone out. Neither of us is the kind of person who first thoroughly looks over a situation before asking herself, "What's in this for me?" That question never comes to mind. So why did instances of guilt plague us while caring for an Alzheimer's patient? It's because of the same reason all other caregivers experience guilt—*every caregiver is an individual with personal rights*—an individual who begins to lose that precious personal identity through the constant caring for another human being.

Having a sense of identity is not the same as having an egotistical, self-absorbed sense of self. These are two completely separate concepts. The first is a realization that you are an independently responsible individual who has uniqueness and God-given rights. The second is a fascination with self, an absorption with oneself.

Apples and Onions

The first recognizes that you have a life and that that life is a *part* of the whole. The second perceives your life as the *center* of society's whole. Alzheimer's caregivers, particularly the at-home twenty-four-hour caregivers, are placed in the difficult situation of needing to understand the difference between these two types of people, between these two concepts of the self. That understanding is imperative; otherwise guilt arises when the caregiver begins to experience feelings of being selfish just because she/he needs some personal space, or requires some solitude, or is socially parched and thirsts for social contact and outside companionship, or just plain needs a rejuvenating dose of mental normalcy by getting away from the dementia for a time.

These feelings are not generated from selfishness, but from a recognition that these people are, indeed, individuals with normal personal needs for their continuing state of well-being—commonplace and normal human needs that nearly every other individual on the planet requires and has the right to enjoy satisfying.

Achieving privacy in one's home is a given for most. For an Alzheimer's caregiver it can seem like a pie-in-the-sky pipedream. So when a caregiver goes into the bathroom, closes the door, and then has the patient immediately open it and look in, the caregiver feels incredible guilt after she/he snaps back at the patient, "Will you *please* leave me *alone?*"; or comes back with something like, "Were you born in a *barn?* For God's *sake,* give me some *privacy!*" This is what I'm talking about. Don't forget, the lock on that bathroom door had to be removed so the patient couldn't lock him/herself in there and possibly injure him/herself with medicines or nail files.

No matter how impeccable the caregiver is about giving the patient high quality daily care, the constant "shadowing" and the continual verbal abuse issuing forth from the patient will eventually wear one's patience down to a fragile, thread-bare state. Whenever this happens, the caregiver then feels overwhelmed with an incredible flood of guilt over what may have been said as a result of her/his quest for some personal space or as an explosive release of deep, pent-up frustration.

The caregiver is a human being with real emotional sensitivities. The caregiver is a human being who has rights of privacy in his/her own home, the right to a social life, the right to enjoy some much-needed leisure time, the right to talk on the phone without someone standing in front of her listening to every word said, the right to walk through his or her house without someone always close on your heels, the right to personal papers in your desk being left alone and not rifled through, purloined, or destroyed, etc. When the caregiver thinks while sighing, "I want my life back," this doesn't intentionally equate to, "I hate you," or "I want you out of here"; it just means that the caregiver is being deprived of basic human rights and is desperately thirsting for them, is starving for what they once took for granted and so enjoyed.

To be sure, being an Alzheimer's at-home caregiver is a thankless job. Yet, the caregiver doesn't particularly care about receiving any forms of thanks or gratitude because we voluntarily chose the job, knowing full well that the patient's dementia automatically negates the patient's appreciation. So the caregiver is never looking for gratitude or appreciation from the patient. The caregivers understand that these will never be theirs, yet being human beings, they do crave some of those basic human rights that their peers so easily take for granted.

Because being this type of caregiver is an incredibly frustrating job, it's not uncommon for the caregivers to experience moments when they feel that they're losing it—going crazy. As mentioned earlier, most medical professionals will deny that Alzheimer's is associated with the term "craziness." They will not use the term; however, craziness is exactly how a caregiver would quickly refer to their job at times. At times they, too, feel as though they're going crazy with the dementia they've been dealing with, and they have a desperate need to get out among normal people. For the at-home caregiver there is no escape from this dementia. They do not enjoy an end to the eight-hour shift at the mental institution. They do not put on their coats and leave the building to return to a quiet home, where they may play soft music, put up their feet, and look forward to being drawn into a good book or movie. They do not go home and get ready for a date or social outing with friends. They cannot simply leave the house when the spur-of-the-moment urge hits them to take off and go visit a neighbor or go window shopping at the mall. The caregivers are bound to home and patient with invisible ties that can only be broken after prior scheduled arrangements have been made for a respite care person to come and temporarily accept the "passing of the reins" for a few hours.

It is not being selfish to miss and crave one's privacy— the privacy that everyone else enjoys within their own home. It is not self-centered to desire to visit friends, have private conversations while on the phone, get a solid night's sleep, to go for a quiet stroll around your property without someone tailing your every move, or to be able to accept social invitations at will. It is not being self-absorbed to want some solitude for the purpose of meditating, reading, study-ing, or just to simply enjoy the rejuvenating effects brought on by some peaceful, quiet time. And when the at-home caregiver reaches the point when this growing craving for common human rights becomes intolerable, she/he will, more frequently than not, experience deep guilt and feel mortified over having those same simple desires that are often wrongly associated with selfishness.

There is also a strong sense of aloneness connected with the caregivers of patients afflicted with this disease. This is because nobody else wants to hear the caregiver's attempts to talk about his/her day or ongoing experiences with the disease. Nobody wants to be a sounding board, if they think they're going to be hearing what they misinterpret as a "sob" story and will be expected to offer words of sympathy that they don't genuinely feel. Nobody, it seems, wants to hear another's problems or be put in the uncomfortable position of having to gift another with comforting solace or possible solutions. Nobody wants to hear, because the general public does not truly fully understand all the varied ramifications of this mentally debilitating disease. Sadly, most Alzheimer's caregivers have eventually discovered this fact the hard way. This is the reason why so many support groups are springing up. Their members can turn to each other for true understanding, for the sincerest emotional support, and constructive problem-solving techniques.

On the frequent occasions when Mary Belle would happen to be in the throes of one of her delusional states, such as having one of her uncontrollable urges to quickly leave the house for the imagined purpose of getting to her shoe factory or teaching job, and she strode away with determination up the drive, we'd have to go after her. Most of the time when this happened, she could not be easily persuaded to voluntarily return home and, if first using any of her own delusional elements didn't succeed, we'd have to firmly guide her back inside after she became physically combative. Sally and I would position ourselves on either side of her and, holding her arms as gently as possible, we'd have to walk her home as she fought us with every fiber in her body.

An hour later she'd come to me and show me the bruises on her arms.

"*Look!*" she'd spout in my face, "*look* what you *did* to me!"

Guilt? Sure I felt guilt over that. Here was an elderly lady with skin as thin as tissue paper that heavily bruised every time a small, three-pound Yorkie jumped on her lap. Here was an aged woman showing me bruises from my own hands that had to hold her firmly and literally wrestle with her when she physically refused to come out of the woods, or come in out of a blizzard, or off an icy porch in winter. Thankfully, my guilt over instances like those ultimately waned (some) because I had to sit down and give the issue some deeper rational thought. I had to logically analyze the situation that was causing me so much heart anguish. As a result, I realized that when Mary Belle got in those defiantly combative moods, those bruises on her arms were nothing compared to a broken hip or neck that she could've easily sustained, if Sally or I hadn't removed her from the potentially harmful situation that she'd insisted on placing herself in. Was it really *us* who caused those surface bruises or was it Mary Belle *herself* who caused them, by insisting on falling to the ground in one of her "dead weight" ploys when we'd try to get her in out of the rain, or when she tried to bite and dig her nails into us as she fought to stay out in a bitter blizzard with no shoes or coat on? There'd be no bruises if she'd only come willingly and peacefully, if she'd only rationally understood the harmful circumstances we were attempting to extract her from. Yet . . . even though the logic of that is sound, I still felt guilt over the fact that those bruises were caused by us. Sometimes, intellectually *knowing* the guilt is a false one doesn't help very much. It still moves over your mind like a long, afternoon shadow silently gliding over a high mountain pond.

As an aside to the above example of unwarranted caregiver guilt, add a trip to the doctor's office into this mix—a trip scheduled for the day following the combative incident, when Mary Belle dramatically extends her bruised arm to nurse, doctor, and anyone who will look, and proclaims in a loud voice, "See what *Mary* did to me?" You have absolutely no idea how that feels. No idea. None. You want to sink into the crack between the floor tiles because, nowadays, the first thing outsiders think of is . . . abuse! Luckily, Mary Belle's doctor and staff were fully familiar with her false accusations, delusions, and other clinical behavioral traits of her disease. Yet, this had happened when Sally had taken her mother into a hospital emergency room. For a daughter who loves her mother, the feeling of having that mother accuse you of physical abuse is beyond description. To say it's devastating doesn't even come close. The pain of it is beyond description. Especially when you've continually done so much, put up with so much, lost so much, voluntarily given up so much, and gone far beyond the call to give your loved one a safe, healthy, and loving environment in which to live out their days.

Sally is one of the most emotionally strong individuals I've ever known. She has the constitution of ten people, yet, on rare occasions, I've seen even *her* retreat to the basement or take off into the forest to have a good, long cry. This was usually caused by a buildup of frustration. Having an Alzheimer's patient in one's home every hour of the day and night can be incredibly frustrating, because there is no personal respite from the unpredictable and abusive behavior. There is no respite from the dirty looks, no escape hatch for extricating oneself from the mean-spirited comments; no magic potion that removes the necessity of having to continually watch over another person so they don't do anything to harm themselves. There's no one but you . . . no one else but you to clean the smeared feces off the television screen or wall, nobody but you to steam clean the new pool of urine from the carpet and give your loved one another shower as, all the while, she fights you tooth and nail.

One of the best examples of a caregiver's frustration came early on, during the time when Mary Belle still had mostly lucid moments. Since Mary Belle loved fish, Sally had decided to take the extra time and effort to treat her mother to a very special "mountain cabin" dinner. She'd set her alarm so she could arise early and sneak off with her fishing gear to spend the morning at her favorite hidden fishing hole. She returned home with a gleaming smile on her face. She had four large rainbow trout and busily spent the afternoon in the kitchen preparing fancy side dishes. I'd set the table and decorated it with fresh-picked wildflowers and a couple of lit tapers. We were going all out to treat Mary Belle to a real Rocky Mountain specialty.

When all was ready and the ambient dining mood was perfect, Sally announced that dinner was ready.

Mary Belle came into the small dining area, slowly scanned the table with a critical eye, and flatly refused to eat because . . . "it wasn't served on her lap in her living room recliner." She then spun on her heels to return to that awaiting recliner.

In total frustration, Sally picked up Mary Belle's loaded plate, marched it into the living room and, without hesitation, dropped it at her mother's feet before striding out the back door, slamming it behind her with a thunderous boom.

I felt Sally's pain so deeply that I was stunned into inaction.

From the living room I heard her mother talking. The sound jarred me out of my numbed state. Unfazed, Mary Belle had released a long, drawn-out, sigh of disgust before promptly addressing her dog. "Tsk-tsk, Molly. For *shame!* Why, just *look* at that *mess!* That mean lady needs to come back here and clean up her mess! I wasn't even hungry anyway. Nobody even bothered to *ask* me if I was hungry. The *nerve* of some *people* around here!"

My heart bled for my friend. I felt so bad for her that I wanted to go run after her to console her, but knew that she was the type who wanted to be alone in times like those to regain her composure. She's like that—she'd rather be alone in situations when she needed to quickly pull herself back together. I respected that.

Sally hadn't been gone for more than three minutes. When she'd returned I'd begun the cleanup. She said that she needed to do it herself. She went straight for the cleaning solutions and attended to the stained carpet in front of Mary Belle's chair. I busied myself elsewhere by clearing the table, blowing out the tapers, and storing the uneaten food for another day. Naturally, nobody felt like eating any more.

While Sally stewed over the incident all evening, Mary Belle acted as though nothing out of the ordinary had happened, and I spent the night quietly tiptoeing around them both. Later that evening, after Mary Belle had retired, Sally felt guilt over her loss of temper, over losing her usual firm grip on her patience and reserve—her logic and rationale. I reminded her that she was not made of granite, that everyone has limits they can be shoved past. I talked about the buttons everyone has that others often stand in front of and repeatedly push.

I'm not sure that all my reasoning worked that night to help her feel less guilty. I think they did. But the Alzheimer's caregiver, especially the at-home caregiver, has to truly realize and thoroughly understand that they're human.

As caregivers we must accept our non-perfection, have no false guilt for not being perfect . . . for not being a saint. We are not unemotional robots.

Throughout the weeks of writing this book and, ultimately, those weeks spent doing an entire rewrite, the rationale of my own mind knew that it was absolutely necessary to relay and document the many symptomatic behavioral examples of Alzheimer's clinical signs that we personally experienced, in order for the book to accurately convey those commonly exhibited elements of the disease, and for the purpose of providing comprehensive information for the general reader. Yet my heart ached every few days when my overly scrupulous conscience kept rudely invading my work by shouting, "Tattletale! Tattletale!" and I'd be forced to take breaks from the documentation to inhale deep breaths of mountain air and get my perspective back in line.

I felt guilt.

I felt as though I were telling tales on this little, white-haired woman. I felt as if I was betraying her in some way. I can't even imagine how Sally must've felt, as she read each new chapter after it was created and then offered suggestions, or reminded me of additional behavioral examples I should include.

What helped me to relieve those guilt pangs was to realize that the cause of my guilt was the uniquely specific "effects" of the disease—those of increasing mental dysfunction. If I'd been writing about most any other type of disease, I'd probably be detailing *physical* symptoms and their resulting problematical ramifications for the primary caregiver. But because Alzheimer's is a disease of the mind—dementia—the symptoms are *behavioral*.

I can't help that.

Mary Belle couldn't help that.

And neither can her daughter.

Nobody can.

So, with this fact in mind, perspective for writing this book returned to its proper place and I was able to continue documenting with a lesser amount of false guilt pangs whispering in my ear. Yes, they still came. They came because I respected Mary Belle. I respected and admired all she'd accomplished throughout her long life and I was writing about her behavior that was now more like a spoiled two-year-old. Such was the raw and glaring fact of the disease's effects and, although I'd previously written and published more than twenty-two books prior to this one, *Love Never Sleeps* was undeniably the absolute hardest to pen in terms of emotional attachment—no contest.

Everyone has feelings. Human emotions are precious blessings to cherish. Our sensitivities do not always make us selfish; they are the powerful impetus behind deep compassion, ecstatic joy, overwhelming generosity, and unconditional love. Although some people seem to use the phrase, "I'm only human," as a catchall excuse to explain away the reasons for their less-favorable actions, with respect to the Alzheimer's caregivers' issue of false guilt, it's a *reason*. They are human. They have human sensitivities. They are not automatons, who never experience feelings of frustration and are beyond having a sense of futility visit them. They are not so insensitive as to never feel twinges of guilt over their temporary loss of temper or patience when pushed beyond their limit. Their thirst for solitude, the right to experience an hour of serenity, privacy, etc., are not the sole rights of the self-absorbed.

Guilt. Guilt is something an unscrupulous, insensitive, unethical individual will never be plagued with. But, for those who care about their behavior and manner of interaction with others, for those whose hearts hold a wellspring of love within, guilt will be an ever-present shadow moving across their conscience. Understanding this goes a long way in helping the Alzheimer's caregivers toward accepting their occasional bouts when the pangs of guilt spear their minds and hearts. As sensitive human beings, we all want to behave in a manner that never emotionally injures another. As sensitive human beings, we feel guilt whenever we think we may have behaved in a less-than-stellar manner toward another. As human beings we have to accept ourselves as we are, and that means that we have to recognize that we *must* care for our own emotional state of being before we can even think about being halfway ready for or qualified to care for another's. Attending to this prerequisite is not being selfish, it's being smart. It's smart to realize that guilt can be a superficial or false emotional response to certain situations in life. It's wise to understand that, as a human being, you have emotional sensitivities—you have feelings too.

The Alzheimer's caregivers show great wisdom when they break through the false guilt barrier by making the realization that they, too, have basic rights as a human being. They have the right to not expect perfection of themselves. They have the right to privacy. They have the right to a social life. They have a right to an identity. They have the right to leisure time, and to a good night's sleep. They have the right to get out with friends. They have a right to lose their patience now and again, to feel a sense of frustration. They have the right to have time to attend to their own personal and business affairs. They have a right to have sympathetic sounding boards without being perceived as someone trying to have a pity-party. They have a right to receive support. They have a right to feel frustrated and have thoughts of regret—all without . . . guilt, for *guilt will try to negate these rights; guilt will smother the love that dwells within these rights.*

I've heard it said that, "Being an Alzheimer's caregiver is all about self-sacrifice." I don't agree. I don't agree because, when one truly sacrifices *all* of self in deference to another, what is there *left* of self to offer as service . . . to gift with their love?

In my opinion, I've seen, firsthand, the evidence of the fact that: There is no greater test of one's patience, tolerance, and acceptance than being an at-home Alzheimer's caregiver. I have seen that being an Alzheimer's at-home caregiver is one of the greatest expressions of love one can gift to another—it being a true example of when . . . love never sleeps. And my firsthand observation of this fact is not a mirrored reflection of our own personal experience with the disease; it's from closely listening to the stories from our neighbors, friends, and other folks who've been there before us. None of them had it easy. None of them escaped the experience without being drawn into a tug-of-war with their conscience when it became infiltrated with false guilt and left their hearts tearing with salty droplets of mortification. Yet all of them held firm to their feelings of love. Love brought them through. Love made them stronger, because it proved the fact that it doesn't take a saint, angel, or a superhuman being to be a caregiver. We humans are capable of so much more inner strength than we could ever hope or dream of having. And, sometimes, it takes walking that long mile to convince us that it's so. When the mile has been traversed, we have the time to pause and, upon looking back, are mildly surprised to discover that we've changed . . . for the better. We've discovered an inner strength—a resilient tenacity that we never knew we had.

V. REFLECTIONS UPON THE WATERS OF HINDSIGHT

Reflections

Reflections. Reflections with a view to hindsight. I imagine that this is the place in the story where readers will anticipate discovering the "Ahh-ha! *Now* we come to the *real* truth of it," the place where the caregivers' seemingly altruistic intentions tumble down a few pegs after living X number of years with the day-to-day symptoms of their loved one's Alzheimer's dementia. But *is* there an "Ahh-ha!" in here? Is there one couched somewhere within the following mix of thoughts? Yes and no. The answer is yes and no because our initial criterion for bringing Mary Belle into our home was solely based on asking ourselves the following question: What is the "spiritual" thing to do in this situation? And, over these past years as being caregivers, we've done some powerful philosophical growing through the various experiential lessons learned. Therefore, hindsight has clearly shown that *making the most spiritual choice is not always the best one for all concerned.* That statement holds more pure truth than the ideology we originally based our decision on. Experience has taught us that the perception of what *appears* to be the most "spiritual" choice could be flawed due to myriad extenuating circumstances, multiple qualifying factors, and/or the presence of varied unknowns associated with the overall situation.

With that truth revealed and lesson learned, readers may now exhale their audible sigh of, "Ahh-ha! They *wouldn't* have taken Mary Belle into their home if they'd previously known everything it would ultimately entail!" But, hold on, that wouldn't be an accurate deduction either because our hindsight conclusion has important dual qualifiers. These qualifiers relate to an Us and Others element. The Us portion says, "Yes, we *would* do it all over again," and the Others aspect relates to what other people finding themselves in the position of making this caregiver decision must closely examine before their final choice is made. This is where those "qualifiers" enter in.

You see, with Mary Belle, there were *two* caregivers involved at the outset of the decision-making process—two caregivers who also *both* had separate *home-based* professions. We both worked at making our livings by working out of the home. We were always home (at least one of us was usually here to cover for the other's absence). These two basic lifestyle elements of our specific situation made all the difference in the world when it came to making our initial decision. Consequently, in our situation, doing the "most spiritual" thing wasn't nearly as complex an issue as it can be for most folks. And that's the crux of the whole matter. So I can't make the "doing the most spiritual thing" a blanket axiom. It can't be an all-inclusive statement or flat, determining criterion to base one's decision on. There're far too many loose threads left hanging that need attention. It's not as clear-cut as it seemed to be.

Sure, we'd all like to live our lives basing decisions on doing whatever the most spiritual choice is, but that choice isn't always that crystal clear. It may appear to be. It may seem to be incredibly obvious, yet that crystal can be clouded with any number of concealed occlusions that escape the naked eye.

Fortunately, we didn't really have to wait until Mary Belle's passing to see what a clear hindsight view would end up looking like. Its reflection shone bright and was sharply outlined while she was still with us. Although after she passed we knew we'd have to replace the bedroom carpeting and refurbish or replace the furniture she destroyed during her irrational illness, we still held firmly to our conclusion—we'd do it all over again. We would. We definitely would. However, there's a great, glaring urgency that I feel compelled to include here, and that is the most important qualifier of all—that of love. I don't want to give the impression that the idea of "love never sleeping" solely applies to those who make the decision to bring an afflicted loved one into their home. I'm not saying that, nor has it ever been my intention to imply it.

I repeat, there were two of us here. Two of us who worked out of the home. Hindsight reveals this as being a highly unusual set of life circumstances which made our decision-making process far less complicated than those confronting most folks faced with this same caregiving decision. My bottom line point here is this: *One's depth of Love is not the determining criterion for decision-making.* This is so important to understand—to truly understand. It's probably the most important concept for a potential caregiver to grasp and take into first consideration, because a decision to place one's loved one in a medical facility instead of bringing them into one's home has *nothing* to do with the depth of love (or lack thereof) they have for their loved one. *Making the nursing home choice does not equate to a lack of love.* I can't overstress this truism. I can't overemphasize this fact, because too many good and deeply compassionate people are too often plagued with guilt when making the medical facility choice. They feel as though they've failed their loved one if they place him/her in a facility. Their conscience is time and again speared with mortifying pangs of guilt generated by painful ideas of abandonment—that they've abandoned their loved one in his/her most desperate time of need. Not so. Not so at all. Not in the least.

There are those people who believed they did the right thing by taking an Alzheimer's-afflicted loved one into their homes and then relocated them into a facility after the disease progressed far enough that personal caregiving was no longer viable for one reason or another. Still, these same caring individuals were assailed with all manner of guilt over not being able to carry their initial decision through to the end. That's the ultimate sampling of the clinically recognized symptom of caregiver's false guilt—that's the quintessential example. It's false because the individual did all in his/her power to remain true to intentions, yet the unforeseen appearance of multiple extenuating circumstances encroached on the original situation and then clearly became the determining factor in taking an alternate road.

We are not all-seeing beings. Life is mutable. Life is an hour-by-hour journey through a land of possibilities—possibilities and potentialities that are most often unforeseen and some, to be sure, undreamed of.

Courses and currents shift.

One's surrounding landscape can alter in a blink of a barn owl's eye.

The once solid ground one could always depend on for being predictable and bringing a sense of security can suddenly liquefy beneath her/his feet.

We take one day at a time and keep an eye on the one predictable axiom in life—Life is Ever-changing—and then, with acceptance, go with the flow of the new current to make the best of the altered course.

Old course or new, what remains as the grounding factor is our love. Whether our lifestyle elements are conducive to caring for a loved one in our home atmosphere, or placing them in a medical facility, has no bearing on the depth or measure of our love. We love that person just the same, no matter which choice is made. And, besides trying to help the public become more knowledgeable in regard to what to expect from an Alzheimer's-afflicted loved one, the point of this book is to emphasize that, no matter what your decision, your love for your loved one will never sleep. If placing them in a nursing home is the only viable solution, then it doesn't mean that your love for them suddenly dozed off and took a long nap. Quite the contrary, it means that, no matter how much false guilt you may experience for making that choice, your love for them never faltered. In your heart you know that . . . love never sleeps.

Postscript

Mary Belle's understanding of the spoken word diminished markedly. Rarely was our presence acknowledged anymore. She began a new routine of repeating a single tearful request, "Daddy, oh, Daddy, please take me home." Day and night the plea echoed through the house. The refrain never altered as her single-minded thought held sway over all others.

Mary Belle's food intake began to decline markedly around the middle of December. We would sit with her and attempt every ruse we could think of to get her to eat a few nourishing bits of protein. Hand-feeding was met with a mouth clamped tightly shut and energetic shakes of the head. What she was eager to eat was goodies, so Sally baked her cheesecakes and I attempted to make them even more attractive by dribbling caramel or chocolate syrup over her generous slice and topping it with pecans. This was eaten with relish. Pies and breakfast sweet rolls were a hit. But then even her gusto for goodies waned, and the desserts were left untouched. We resorted to giving her a variety of those specialized, high-nutrient drinks along with an assortment of fruit juices. And then those were left alone or dumped on the floor.

The week before Christmas Sally and I came down with the flu. Having to still take care of Mary Belle, we did our best to avoid prolonged contact with her in order to try to spare her the possibility of contracting it. Three days before Christmas, she showed the symptoms we were hoping to avoid seeing in her. She'd begun having diarrhea and vomiting. Since she was refusing fluids, we were afraid of her experiencing the same dehydration that we had. On Christmas Eve day we decided she required fluids, and getting her down to a hospital in our truck was out of the question, so we called an ambulance. The drive down the mountain pass was an hour long.

Once at the hospital, Sally accompanied her mother into the emergency exam room while I sat out in the waiting room. We were there for six hours. Sally had to argue with the doctor to get him to hydrate Mary Belle with an I.V. drip. The nurse had a difficult time getting the line in due to Mary Belle's fragile skin and veins. A large hematoma developed at the site. Sally fought to have her mother admitted, yet we ended up bringing Mary Belle back home with us because the doctor claimed that "the patient didn't meet the admittance criteria for Medicare." Sally wanted to know what that had to do with anything, since Mary Belle had an excellent Aetna health insurance policy. It seemed that, for the elderly, medical care facilities viewed Medicare as the primary insurance no matter what additional health policies a patient had. Sally was furious. Her hands were tied. Her mother had come in the ambulance with no shoes or coat and we were expected to take her home that way in frigid winter weather. The hospital offered their patient a pair of little socks to wear to the car and a blanket to wrap around Mary Belle against the biting wind. The blanket was the one Mary Belle had urinated on. Sally told them they could keep it and took her coat off and wrapped it about her mother. We drove home in silence—Sally too infuriated to even speak.

Because Sally and I were still dealing with our own flu symptoms, we'd had to call off the Christmas party we'd planned for family and friends and cancel our attendance at my daughter's family gathering. So, on Christmas night my daughter came by for a few hours with my granddaughter. During their stay we heard a loud thump from Mary Belle's room. Sally raced upstairs to find her mother had fallen. She was on the floor with her slacks over her head, arms shoved up the pant legs, and nothing else on. We checked her over and got her back up. Nothing seemed to be broken. We felt we had lucked out.

The following day, Mary Belle exhibited dramatic signs of having had a stroke. She could no longer stand erect, her speech was slurred, her vision wasn't as focused as before, and she developed a new restlessness of pacing the room and calling out more desperately to Daddy.

On December 30th, she stopped all intake of fluids.

On January 3rd, Mary Belle took to her bed and Sally called her brother and sister. She informed them of their mother's declining state and suggested that they might want to come see her before she got any worse. Tony immediately made arrangements to fly out and stayed with us for four days. We all took turns sitting with Mary Belle. Sally spent time dripping water into her mother's mouth, coating her lips with Vaseline, and doing whatever she could to attend to her and make her as comfortable as possible. During one lucid moment when Mary Belle's mind broke through the cloudy drifts of her semi-comatose state, she focused her eyes on Tony and whispered, "My son, my baby." She managed to do the same for Sally when she looked up at her, smiled, and squeezed her hand as if to acknowledge a promise kept.

On January 5th, Mary Belle's pupils became unresponsive. Sally and I never left her side. There was always one of us with her. We either sat on the bed with her and stroked her hand or forehead, or we lay beside her with our arms around her. We kept talking softly to her. "Daddy's in the Light, Mary Belle. Look for the Light, it's Home. Take Daddy's hand when you see him reaching out to you. The

Light's Home, Mary Belle. It's warm and safe." Sally and I spelled one another during the night hours so at least one of us got a few hours' sleep.

On the morning of January 8th, the day after Tony left, Sally was on the telephone with one of her nurse friends while I was upstairs sitting on the bed with Mary Belle. Her breathing suddenly changed from labored and moaning to soft and quiet. I called for Sally. She was stroking Mary Belle's forehead when her mother took three more soft breaths before her Daddy took her Home. She went home on his birthday.

Sally lay sobbing with her arm around her mother. "My mama's gone," she softly cried. "My mama's gone." I curled behind Sally with my arm over her. So helpless feeling, so heartrending, so deep the pain.

An hour later Sally called 911. Six sheriff deputies arrived at the house to look over the scene. They didn't take more than a couple of minutes to determine that the death was a natural one. The deputies were all very kind and sympathetic. A few stayed behind until the coroner arrived. She had no problems with the situation and "called" the time of death, making an additional note to record the 8:37 time, when we said the last breath had been taken.

After the coroner and deputies left and Sally and I were again alone in the cabin, we returned to Mary Belle's room. Sobbing the whole time, we carefully removed her clothing. With the greatest love and respect we gently washed her, anointed her with some myrrh oil, and dressed her in her favorite clothes before calling the mortuary.

Two hours later, the mortuary gentlemen arrived. They were extremely kind and soft-spoken. They treated Mary Belle with the highest regard. As we watched their van slowly move up our drive and disappear into the dense shadows of the piney forest, I completely lost it. It was then that I'd realized that losing Mary Belle had been like losing my own mother. And, together, Sally and I clung to each other and cried long and hard for the loss of "our" mother.

Neither of us has a single regret. Sally kept true to her promise to never put her mother into a nursing home and I've kept my promise to document Mary Belle's disease.

This book is not mine, it's Mary Belle's. It's her legacy, born of a wish to bring greater knowledge and understanding about Alzheimer's to the world. No, this is not my book at all . . . it's all Mary Belle's.

A Tribute to Mary Belle – A Lady

Independent Woman
Loving Wife at Age 31
Attentive Mother of 3
Favored Girl Scout Leader
Cub Scout Den Mother
Accomplished Square Dancer
Supportive Sports Mom
Loving Grandmother
Avid Golfer
Pool Shark
Ace Bowler
Baseball Fan (Royals)
Turkey Shoot Champion
Camper Extraordinaire
Ping-Pong Expert
Eager Church Activities Participant
Professional Tax Accountant
World Traveler
Public Speaker
Widow at Age 56
Independent Woman Again
Alzheimer's

A Daughter's Afterword

Looking back, I believe I've found evidence of the first signs of Mary Belle's Alzheimer's fifteen years ago. She had always prepared friends' tax returns and back in 1986, she started asking folks to find another accountant, as she was having trouble with the calculations. This is a slowly developing insidious disease that is almost impossible to detect in its early stages. Watching my mother through these years I've come to believe that the hardest part for her was the two- or three-year period when she knew her mind was failing. She was helplessly frustrated and quietly terrified. She had seen what Alzheimer's had done to some of her friends.

Never will Mary Belle and I be able to fully express our gratitude and thanks to Mary Summer Rain. There are not enough words, hugs, or tears. Without Rain's financial support, emotional strength, and generosity I would not have been able to care for Mom at home. I'm sure that Mary Belle knew what she was saying when she called Rain "Saint Mary" and that was exactly what she meant. I concur.

369

Mary Belle's husband, Rudy, endured several rounds of experimental chemotherapy, all the while knowing that it would do nothing to help him—his hope was that perhaps it would help in the research to benefit future generations. This book has been a joint effort of Mary Summer Rain, Mary Belle, and myself. At first Mom had some qualms about people "reading about her," but she saw past her personal privacy issues in the hope that this book would benefit you or your loved ones. As a daughter I could not be more proud of my mother as I share those privacy issues. Mary Belle gave her love constantly in life to all those who were fortunate enough to have known her and continues to give through this book.

Mary Belle's grandmother lived to enjoy the wonderful age of 92. Mary Belle herself saw 82. She had "very good" medical insurance with a well-known and long-established, nationwide company. This insurance company has, time and again, paid a full 80 percent of all her medical expenses without fail or contest. However, while I was reading the fine print of the insurance policy I discovered to my dismay that "dementia" is excluded from the coverage. Recently, her former employer sent a secondary policy for extended care provisions that they were offering to supplement the original policy. Mary Belle wasn't eligible because her condition was then a "pre-existing" one. This secondary policy would've greatly helped us with the expenses of caring for her either at home or in a nursing home if it hadn't come too late for her. Her primary policy was apparently written in the dark ages when Alzheimer's was still a total medical enigma.

The disease of Alzheimer's caused the physical destruction of my mother's brain cells, just as the malignant brain tumor my father died of also destroyed his brain cells. Dad's illness was covered, Mom's wasn't. I interject this issue for two reasons. To the reader who is a potential caregiver, please do yourself a huge favor now—right now—check over your loved one's insurance policies. It could be a financial lifeline. Secondly, to the reader who may have ties to the insurance industry, I have just one comment . . . it's way past time for some across-the-board changes.

Hampton Roads Publishing Company

. . . for the evolving human spirit

Hampton Roads Publishing Company
publishes books on a variety of subjects,
including metaphysics, health, integrative medicine,
visionary fiction, and other related topics.

For a copy of our latest catalog, call toll-free
(800) 766-8009, or send your name and address to:

Hampton Roads Publishing Company, Inc.
1125 Stoney Ridge Road
Charlottesville, VA 22902

e-mail: hrpc@hrpub.com
www.hrpub.com

So although this "disconnected" late stage of Alzheimer's would appear to mostly consist of behavior completely disassociated from reality, we witnessed sparks of patient recognition that seemed to break through that invisible wall separating her world from ours.

Examples

Up until that point in time, the television had been a wonderful diversion for Mary Belle. She'd sit in her recliner and watch it for hours. Yet, now she'd lost the comprehension that the television was not always a true representation of reality. She couldn't differentiate between the reality of a newscast program and the make-believe of a soap opera or movie. If there was some type of villain on the TV, she'd go up to the screen and bang on it, "You no good, so-and-so. I'm gonna kill you!" At this point, either Sally or I would go upstairs and simply change the channel to a more innocuous type of programming. Mary Belle wouldn't even notice that the change had been made and would sit back down and again be drawn into the action on the screen.

More often than not, though, the television was something to be ignored. As time passed, she would seem to take no heed that it was even on. Her past enjoyment taken from watching it had appeared to wane considerably. Instead of talking to the people on the screen, we'd hear her having a lively conversation, and, when one of us went up to check who she was talking to, she'd have her chair over in front of the closet, talking to the hanging clothing. Other times she'd be conversing with the bedpost. Many times the one-sided discussion would be with her collection of stuffed animals. Although the interest in the television had diminished to nearly nil, we still put it on in the morning for her and didn't shut it off until bedtime.

There was no longer any sign of verbal comprehension when we attempted to engage Mary Belle in a conversation.

Frequently, one of us would go into her room and sit on her bed to spend time with her. She seemed to prefer non-communication rather than being drawn into even the simplest of conversations. We'd like to think that she enjoyed the company, yet would react to such company in a disassociative manner of behavior. She'd forget you were there and talk to the stuffed animals or the television.

When Judy came out to Colorado and stayed a couple of days, she spent most of the time up in her mother's room. Not being able to draw Mary Belle into any logical conversation, she offered her opinion. "I think Mom needs more human contact."

No clue. Absolutely no clue in understanding the extent of Mary Belle's declining mental state. We could spend our entire day with Mary Belle in her room and it'd be as though we weren't even there. We knew this from experience. Being the sole caregivers, we'd taken extra steps to insure that our loved one had plenty of human contact. We were not solely her food delivery people or the maids who only entered the room to vacuum and change the bed. We had spent hours out of our day sitting with her and keeping her company. Yet, evidence of her acknowledging our physical presence was not there. More the contrary, it would always seem as though we were made to feel that we were actually unwelcome in her private domain . . . a presence to be barely tolerated.

Since the enjoyment of the television had waned to almost nothing, Mary Belle would occupy her time with other activities. One in particular was that of stripping her bed down to the mattress . . . three times a day. She'd take off the spread, the blanket, both sheets, the waterproof mattress cover we had to buy, and even the pillowcases. These would be placed in piles about the room, stuffed in desk drawers, or shoved into her toilet chair . . . after she'd used it.

When she initially began taking her bed apart, I'd go in and remake it for her. She'd sit in her recliner and tell me